Templar Alchemy

By Janis Ford

MisterRee Books

Templar Alchemy

Janis Ford

Author: Janis Ford | Editor: Mister Ree

Copyright: © 2015 MisterRee Books

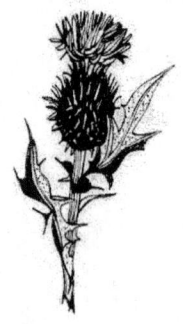

Book Dedication

I would like to give credit and a big heart-felt 'thank you' to Mister Ree Books and The Priory for all their continual support and guidance; for having faith in me and giving me the confidence to build on what I so love doing.

The Priory will always be the cornerstone of my existence and at the heart of whom I truly am.

The ride has been of pure and perfect joy; bumps and laughter in harmony all along the way.

Janis

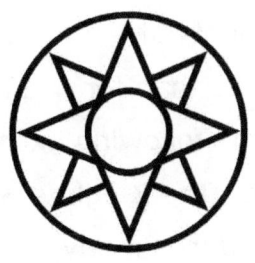

The Star of Ninasu

KNIGHT TEMPLAR ALCHEMY

MAGICAL PRACTICES USING THE SACRED STONES, HERBS AND POTIONS OF THE SERPENT PRIESTHOOD

'When the black flame is lit, man attains to wisdom the nature of Solomon'.

INTRODUCTION

Mankind has always had a connection to this planet and the bounty she produces, apart from food; none more so than for use in magic, health and healing. As the following extract from the opening section of 'The Knight's Bible' explains the earth also produces many poisons, yet also the ant-dote – thus keeping a perfect balance.

When we walk upon this earth as practitioners of magic and healing, right from the very beginning of our earthly journey we acknowledge the many gifts that this planet has to offer and that freedom, fervency and zeal are thus represented by Chalk, Charcoal and Clay. There is nothing freer than Chalk, the slightest touch of which leaves a trace; there is nothing more fervent than Charcoal, for to it, when properly ignited, the most obdurate metals will yield; there is nothing more zealous than Clay, our mother Earth, for it alone of all the elements has never proved unfriendly to man.

Bodies of water deluge mankind with rain, oppresses with hail and drown with inundation; the air rushes in storms and prepares the tempest; the fire lights up the volcano; but the Earth, ever kind and indulgent, is found subservient to mankind's wishes. Though constantly harassed, more to furnish the luxuries than the necessaries of life, she the earth, never refuses her accustomed yield, spreading the pathway of mankind with flowers and the table with plenty.

Though she produces poison, still she supplies the antidote, and returns with interest every good committed to her care; and when at last we are called upon to pass through the dark valley of the shadow of death, she once more receives us, and piously covers our remains within her bosom, thus admonishing us that as from it we came, so to it we must shortly return.

So thus as we gain wisdom and knowledge from the earthly teaching as well as the practices of the Templars, teachings that have their origins way back in time; being hidden in time for many years. Using the abundant herbs and stones of the plain, we are able to move forwards in our daily practices to evolve. The origins of the teachings in this book go way back to the ancient Sumerian times and even beyond when the peoples of the planet were taught magical and healing practices that became lost in time; known down through the years to only a few who protected the wisdom and knowledge for all times, away from the grasp of those who would wish harm. The Knights Templar or Serpent Priesthood, were often known as the 'Keepers of Secrets' and indeed they have protected and guarded their ancient knowledge down through the centuries, until a time such as now, when the secrets can once again be revealed. *Extract taken from 'The Knights Bible'*

'In the forest of destruction I saw an open book.'

CHAPTERS:

- INTRODUCTION
- ALCHEMICAL RECIPE OF CRAFT
- SACRED STONE, HERB AND POTION LISTING
- HEALING WITH SACRED STONES/THE SAMNA EMUA
- SERPENTINE, ARAGONITE, OBSIDIAN AND HOWLITE
- WORKING WITH HERBS: THE SECRET LORE OF ALKA ANTAM
- HEALING WITH THE RAKBU DAG
- NAPARU AND CANDLE MAGIC
- TOURMLINE AND MAGNESITE
- INFINITY TRANCE: THE GENERATION OF LIFE
- MAGNESITE, SUNSTONE AND OPALITE
- REFERENCE FOR SACRED STONE/HERB MAGIC
- VOODOO: A PRACTICAL GUIDE

8

- ⏀ ALCHEMY: AN INTRODUCTION AND GUIDE
- ⏀ HERBAL PREPARATIONS, POUCHES AND CANDLES
- ⏀ A PRACTICAL GUIDE FOR CREATING POTIONS, SPELLS, POUCHES, CANDLES AND LOTIONS ETC:
- ⏀ TRUE BLACK SALT
- ⏀ TO KNOW – TO WILL – TO DARE – TO KEEP SILENT

'When the world forgets Nature, Nature will remind the world'

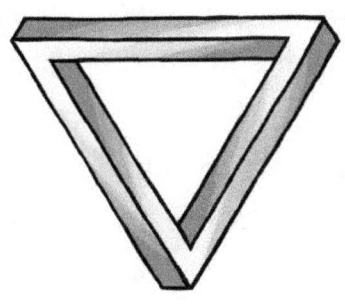

ALCHEMICAL RECIPE OF PERFECT CRAFT

Take one Chalice full of Love and Light
Mix in equal measures of Destiny and Desire.
Carefully pour the mixture over the Cup of Life
And sprinkle in the Sacred Stones of Healing.
To all of which add several large pinches (to
taste) of the Herbs of the Plain.

Blend well together with Dark, Light and Fire.
Next take equal portions of Reverence and Mirth
And whisk well together with Love and Trust until
light and frothy.

Take a sachet each of dried blood, bone, hand
and horn and sift liberally over.

Fold all ingredients smoothly together with the
Sacred Sword of Knowledge, then allow the
mixture to stand for nine minutes until
The Soul fires up and the Spirit raises from
within.

Finally add the Essence of the Universe and bind
as One with the Elixir of Life,
Until the Alchemical Recipe of Perfect Craft has
been created.

'Death is never the end but the beginning'

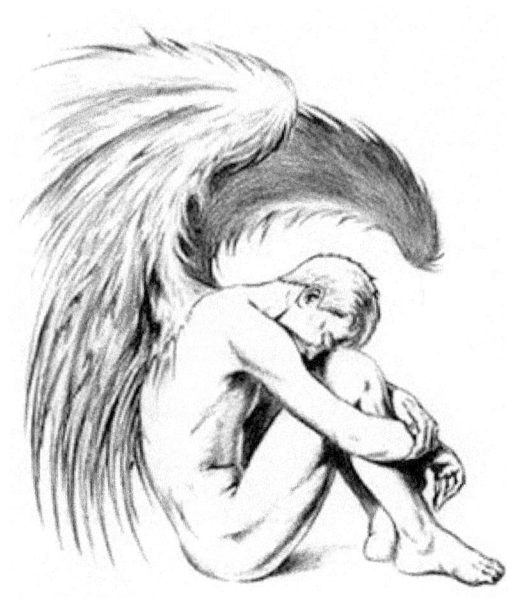

KNIGHT TEMPLAR SACRED STONE, HERB AND POTION LISTING FOR THE PRACTICES OF ALCHEMY

AMBER: Utu – The Sun – Life Giver – South – Grid of Poland

The name of Amber was known as Ambre (Old English), Ambra (Latin), and Anbar Ambergris (Arabic). The colour of Amber varies from yellow to orange with sometimes traces of red, green, blue, violet, and black. Green amber is produced by heat treatment. It is soft and is easily damaged, with a hardness rating of 2.5. It is a fossilized tree resin of ancient pine and conifer trees and is known to have the DNA of extinct species. Although Amber is found in Norway, Denmark and England having been washed to the coast, the purest form is found in Poland.

It is said that the holder will feel happiness and it has been used since 8000 B.C.E, though is not considered to be an anniversary gemstone.

Healing Ability: Eyes, lungs, throat, digestive system, and glandular swellings

Magical Ability: Clarity and insight, life giver, good luck, longevity, attunes magnetic forces, calms aggression, and stimulates mental focus

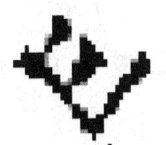

4th House of Utu

<u>OBSIDIAN</u>: Enlil - Venus – Insight – East – Grid of Japan; Kur – Mercury – Underworld – Southwest – Grid of Japan

It is said that this stone was discovered by Obsius in Ethiopia and named after him. This is not to be confused with the purest origin. The colour of Obsidian is black; a natural glass formed by volcanic lava that cooled quickly. Other colours found in Obsidian are: brown, red, blue, grey, and green. Snowflake Obsidian is where there are bubbles or crystals in the stone. Obsidian is relatively fragile, having a hardness rating of 5 and although discovered in Ethiopia, its purest form is in Japan and some date back to 21,000 B.C.E. It is not considered to be an anniversary gemstone, but is used to make mirrors and sacrificial tools

Healing Ability: Realignment of energy, bones, head, and stimulates brain activity

Magical Ability: Insight, underworld travel, and energy stability

1st House of Enlil (Lahmu)

13th House of Kur

TIGER'S EYE: Enki (Arata in higher degrees) – The Earth – The Gift – West – Grid of South Africa

Tiger's Eye was known Cat's Eye, African Cat's Eye, and Crocidolite. The colour is of yellow and golden brown stripes and is chatoyant quartz (has an optical reflectance effect). It is thought to be all-seeing due to its appearance and has a hardness rating of 7; be sure to avoid temperature changes. The purest form is found in South Africa and is given in the 9th year of Handfasting.

Healing Ability: Asthma, kidney, heart disease, psoriasis, and high blood pressure

Magical Ability: Provides comfort to the weak and sick, focuses the mind, and protection during travel

2nd House of Enki (Arata)

MOONSTONE: Nanna – The Moon – Emotion – North – Grid of Sri Lanka

Moonstone is named due to its resemblance to the colour of the Moon. The colour is a soft milk colour and has either a blue or white sheen and has a hardness rating of 6 and is easily scratched. The purest form is found in Sri Lanka and is given in the 13th year of Handfasting.

Healing ability: Aligns vertebrae, assists digestion, fertility, and balances emotion

Magical Ability: Protection, good fortune, and arouses passion

10th House of Nanna (Anshar)

CARNELIAN: Nergal (Anunna in higher degrees) – Mars – Fertility, Initiative – Northwest – Grid of Brazil

Carnelian is also known as cornelian, from the Latin word meaning horn. The colour is from bright orange to reddish orange. Carnelian will be a deeper red dependant on the iron oxide. It is placed in the sun to change any tints to red, and has a hardness rating of 7. The purest form of Carnelian is found in Brazil.

Healing Ability: Headaches, nausea, blood, liver, speech, and infection

Magical Ability: Provides comfort to the weak or sick, enables courage, to cause sudden noise or disturbance. Also for good luck and will empower creativity

8th House of Nergal (8th house of Anunna)

CLEAR QUARTZ: Inanna – Saturn – Sexual – Northeast – Grid of Russia

Quartz is also known as Krustallos, from the Greek word meaning ice. The colour has different names; the transparent quartz is a rock crystal. Brown quartz is known as Smokey quartz; there is a rose quartz and even Amethyst. It is not considered to be an anniversary stone. Quartz has a hardness rating of 7. The purest form of Quartz is found in Russia.

Healing Ability: Nausea, Infection, and sexual problems, lethargy

Magical Ability: Visions of future, raising power, and cleansing space

3rd House of Inanna

BLUE LACE AGATE: Namtar – Neptune – Communication – Southeast - Grid of Egypt

The agate was named after the river Achates, now the Drillo, in Sicily. Agate comes in most colours. Blue agate is as expected, light blue. Moss agate is dark green, often with clear patches. Tree agate is green and white. Agate is porous, so is usually dyed to enhance its natural colour, and it has a hardness rating of 7 and is given in the 12th year of Handfasting. The purest form of Agate is found in Egypt

Healing Ability: Damaged skin, reawakens cell tissue, rash, general skin infection, soothes discomfort, arthritis, bones, pancreas, blood sugar balance, bites, and stings

Magical Ability: Communication, raising power, to defeat enemies, and protection during travels

6th House of Namtar (Ea)

AMETHYST: Martu – Nibiru – Wisdom All – Cortex – Grid of India

The name Amethyst was known as Amatist (Old English), Amethystus (Latin), and Amethustos (Greek). The colour Is Purple, Lilac, or Mauve, but the highest quality is transparent. It has a hardness rating of 7 and is given in the 4th and 6th year of Handfasting.

Amethyst is heat treated to produce Citrine

Healing ability: Psychic ability, brain activity, strengthens immunity, purifies the blood, headaches, and blood sugars

Magical Ability: Aids drunkenness (either positive of negative), love charms, protection against theft, calms sleep, enables travel in dream state, insight to solve problems, raise energy, charge soul and body, and enhances spirituality.

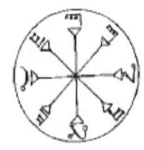

7th House of Martu

<u>FIRE OPAL</u>: Ishkur – Jupiter – Stability – Hidden North – Grid of Mexico

The name opal is known as Upala (Sanskrit), Opallios (Greek), and Opalus (Latin), meaning precious stone. Opal comes in most colours. Fire Opal is known as Mexican Fire Opal as it is there the purest form can be found. The purest form of Fire Opal is found in Mexico

Healing Ability: Heart, feet, hands, circulation, and muscular

Magical Ability: Attunes to higher plains, heightens awareness, used during the Crowning Ceremony.

꜌꜍꜎

11th House of Ishkur

JASPER: Resheph – Mars – Protection – Hidden East – Grid of Germany

The name Jasper was known as Iaspis (Greek), the colour of Jasper is red, brown, green, greyish-blue, and yellow. Often jasper is multi-colour and has a hardness rating of 7. The purest form of Jasper is found in Germany

Healing Ability: Stomach, gynaecological problems, depression,

Magical Ability: Brings joy and drives away those who attack

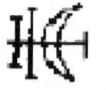

HEMATITE: Ereshkigal – Pluto – Negative Existence – Hidden West; Ninlil – Uranus – Positive Existence – Hidden South. Both are of the Grid of North America

The name Hematite is also known as Haematite, from the haem name for blood (Greek). In ancient times Hematite objects were made and placed in tombs. The colour of Hematite has the appearance of silvery metal, but when in ground, turns to a red powder as if it were bleeding. It has a hardness rating of 6.5. Hematite occurs in a soft, fine-grained, earthy form called red ochre or ruddle. Intermediate between these types are compact varieties, often with a reniform surface (kidney ore) or a fibrous structure (pencil ore). Red ochre is used as a pigment in paints and crayons, a purified form, rouge, is used to polish plate glass.

Healing Ability: Hysteria, bladder, venereal disease, and strengthens body.

Magical Ability: General healing, resistance to life's stress, inspires inner life, keeps inward peace

9th House of Ereshkigal (Anu)

LAPIS LAZULI: Nammu – Universal Intelligence – Hidden Grid of Afghanistan

The name Lapis comes from the Spanish word for pencil. It is also known as Laurite. The colour of Lapis Lazuli is shades of blue, some with speckled veining of white (Calcite) or yellow (Pyrite). However, the finest quality had little or no veining from other elements. It was used for cosmetics and painting and buried with the dead to guide them towards the L.i.g.h.t. It is given in the 7th and 9th year of Handfasting.

Healing Ability: Increase abilities, fever, negative emotions

Magical Ability: Clarity and insight, life giver, good luck, longevity, attunes magnetic forces, calms aggression, and stimulates mental focus

Intelligence of Nammu 'Success and Protection'

SERPENTINE: With One – Spiritual Connection – Hidden Site of England

The name Serpentine was named due to its colour and marking similar to that of a snake. It has a direct connection to all that is spiritual both on the plain and in time itself. It was used for both positive and negative practice, being of purpose in time and travel. It is given in the 12th Degree of Grand Craft and developed within the Degree of Magus.

Healing Ability: Absorbs negative emotions, reflects negative patterns in the biochemistry, and is able to regulate the hypothalamus.

Magical Ability: Blocks negative thought, reflects negative thought, tunes to the frequency of Spirituality, Blocks Attackers on a Magical Level, and is able to raise the seal of 333.

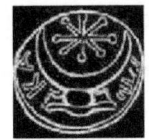

ARAGONITE: Shupa – Pluto – Guardian – West – Grid of Spain. Church of St. Mary – Guadalajara – Spain

The name Guadalajara derives from the Arab name, meaning 'River of Stones'. Aragonite is a carbonate mineral and colours vary from colourless, white, grey, yellow-white, and reddish-brown. The composition of Aragonite is 40% calcium, 13% Carbon, and 47% Oxygen. It is soft and is easily damaged, with a hardness rating of 3.5. Although it is best sourced from Aragon in Spain (Where it name was given), it may be further sourced from Morocco, France, Sicily, England (Cumbria), United States, and Mexico. It is said that the holder will obtain future insight.

Healing Ability: Warms, brings energy to entire body, muscle spasms, calcium absorption, and physical perfection.

Magical Ability: Grounding, focus of thought, visualisation, discipline of the mind, and future insight.

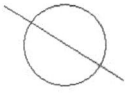

Shupa – Pluto R.O.S.E Magnetic

HOWLITE: Anshar – Moon – Damuzi Existence – North – Grid of America - Old Faithful Geyser, Calistoga – California – America

Howlite can be green, white, or blue. A calming stone and if placed on the 'inner mind' or rather the third eye, it can assist with travelling outside the body to past, present and the future. It is named after Henry How, a geologist from Nova Scotia (New Scotland in Canada – In Latin). A hardness rating of 3.5, its general composition is of calcium silicoborate and is commonly dyed to imitate other gems, such as Turquoise and Lapis Lazuli.

Healing Ability: Insomnia, stress, calcium levels, teeth, bones and purifying blood.

Magical Ability: Travelling out of the body, of memory, knowledge and progress. It will cleanse the Aura.

Anshar – Moon R.O.S.E Magnetic

TOURMALINE: Nammu – Universal – Purification – Protection – Energy - Sacred Number 9 – Yellow - Brazil

Tourmaline is an electromagnetic mineral that if rubbed will rejuvenate its magnetic impulse time and time again. The common colour of Tourmaline is black, but further variations are green, bicoloured, or even multicoloured. The purest source is found in Brazil and it has an average hardness rating of 7.5.

Healing Ability: Assists the body's energy distribution, central nervous system, strengthens thought, and encourages well being

Magical Ability: Protects against unwanted energies, reduces fear and obsessions, aids inspiration and understanding, and is able to promote love and friendship. Further used during purification rituals

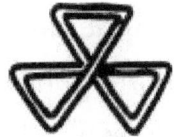

Intelligence of Nammu 'Success and Protection'

DARK AMBER: Ar – The Sun – Life Giver – South – Grid of Poland

The name of Amber was known as Ambre (Old English), Ambra (Latin), and Anbar Ambergris (Arabic). The colour of Amber varies from yellow to orange, and sometimes had traces of red, green, blue, violet, and black. Green amber is produced by heat treatment. It is soft and is easily damaged, with a hardness rating of 2.5. It is a fossilized tree resin of ancient pine and conifer trees and is known to have the DNA of extinct species. Although Amber is found in Norway, Denmark and England and has been washed to the coast, the purest form is found in Poland. It is said that the holder will feel happiness and has been used since 8000 B.C.E, though is not considered to be an anniversary gemstone.

Healing Ability: Eyes, lungs, throat, digestive system, and glandular swellings

Magical Ability: Clarity and insight, life giver, good luck, longevity, attunes magnetic forces, calms aggression and stimulates mental focus.

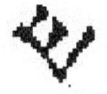

AZURITE: Kishar – Jupiter – Strength – North – Grid of America - Tequiquiapan Volcanic Springs – Grid of Mexico

Also found in Otavi, Namibia; the name for Azurite originates from a Persian term, meaning 'blue'. Colours range from light blue to dark blue to almost black. A Hardness rating of 3.5 - 4, its general composition is 55 % copper, 37 % oxygen, 7 % carbon, and 1 % hydrogen.

Healing Ability: Spleen, thyroid and arthritis.

Magical Ability: Activates expansion of consciousness, stimulates psychic abilities, clearer meditation, enhances inspiration, and assists with mental control.

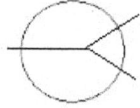

Kishar – Jupiter R.O.S.E Magnetic

MAGNESITE: Ilu – G-O-D – Universe – Peace – Passion – Focus - Northwest to South – Sacred Number 3 – Black Spirits – Grid of Brazil

Magnesite (magnesium Carbonate) has the same crystal structure as Calcite (Calcium carbonate). It is often dyed to resemble turquoise. The common colour of Magnesite is white, but can further be white with grey lines, tinted yellow or brown. It can also be transparent. For centuries the Native Americans crafted Magnesite into jewellery, and further used it as a form of currency. The purest source is found in Brazil and it has an average hardness rating of 4 - 4.5.

Healing Ability: Assists the body's energy distribution, awakens the metabolism, lowers cholesterol, calms headaches and migraines, calms stomach cramps, strengthens bones and teeth, and assists regular rhythm of blood-flow

Magical Ability: Helps to bring peace, stimulates passion, and is able to promote focus when travelling either within the earthly plain, or other plains. Helps to protect against false love and false friends, further used during Rites of Passage

Associations: Aragonite, Dolomite, Strontianite, Calcite, and Serpentine

Sacred Locations: Brazil, Austria, China, Korea, America, and some places within Europe

Other Names: White Turquoise, Green Turquoise, Marshmallow Turquoise, Lime Turquoise, Chalk Turquoise, and Mojave.

Ilu – 'Black Spirits'

SUNSTONE: Amalug – Goddess – Creator – Existence – Protector – Love - Northeast to South – Sacred Number 9 – White Spirits – Grid of Norway

Sunstone is a variety of 'feldspar', meaning that it is formed from a group of minerals that are required in the formation of rocks; namely, types of aluminium silicate with calcium, potassium, sodium or barium. Significant feldspar is moonstone. Sunstone is a reddish brown or golden colour, with colour strands red, orange, yellow and green, which are caused by inclusions of goethite or hematite. The purest source is found in Tvedestrand south Norway and it has an average hardness rating of 6 - 6.5.

Healing Ability: Lifts depression, reduces stress, enhances physical and sexual energy, good for use with SAD (Seasonal Affective Disorder), treatment of stomach ulcers, digestive problems, and excess weight

Magical Ability: Dispels fears and phobias, enhances leadership qualities to the holder, reflects psychic attacks, enhance life-force energy, encourages optimism/enthusiasm. Placed next to a white candle it will spread protective energies throughout a building

Direct Associations: Dark Amber, Azurite, Howlite, Quartz, Hematite, Tiger's Eye, Moonstone, Lapis Lazuli, and Tourmaline

Other Associations: Adventurine Feldspar, Aventurine Feldspar, Aventurine Orthoclase, and Heliolite

Sacred Locations: Norway, Siberia, and the United States of America

Amulug – 'White Spirits

OPALITE (OPAL): The Me – Inner Self – Green Man – Mugwort - Number 60 – Red Spirits – Grid of Australia

Opalite resembles Opal and is commonly used in jewellery. It is a synthetic mineral and is highly energetic. There are distinct connection to all forms of Opal within the magical sequence, and the aspects of the Hidden Knowledge. The main Opal source is found in Coober Pedy in South Australia and is considered to have healing properties, thus its classification as a Sacred Stone

Healing Ability: Calms temper, stabilises nerves, alleviates depression, enhances sexual drive and experience, assists transition in life, brings peace, purifies blood, and purifies kidneys

Magical Ability: Enhances psychic powers, reflection of thoughts, focuses visualisation, assists communication and interpretation, encourages telepathy, enhances channelling, and removes energy blockages

Direct Associations: Obsidian, Jasper, Azurite, dark Amber, and Sunstone

Other Associations: Opal fluorite, Opalized fluorite, Tiffany stone, Ice Cream Opalite, Purple Opal, Sea opal, Bertrandite

Sacred Locations: Hong Kong, Australia, Mexico, Brazil, Ethiopia, and the United States of America

MALACHITE: Absorption of Knowledge – Grid of Siberia

Malachite is a semi-precious stone and its colour is green, used as an ornamental and gemstone, its main source is located in Siberia. Egyptians record the earliest mining of this stone as around 4000 BCE.

Healing Ability: Assists sleep patterns, calms nervous system, and boosts energy levels

Magical Ability: Worn as a pendant to protect from negative magical forces, warns of trouble, balances emotion, calms the life cycle, and assists with the absorption of knowledge

SMOKEY QUARTZ: **Visualisation – Grid of Scotland**

Quartz is also known as Krustallos, from the Greek word meaning ice. The colour has different names; the transparent quartz is a rock crystal, Brown quartz is known as Smokey quartz. There is a Rose quartz and even Amethyst. It is not considered to be an anniversary stone. Quartz has a hardness rating of 7. The purest form of Smokey Quartz is found in Scotland.

Healing Ability: Nausea, infection, and sexual problems, lethargy

Magical Ability: Visions of future, raising power and cleansing space

<u>ONYX:</u> **Psychic Attack – Grid of Brazil**

Onyx is a name that means 'ring' (Originally an Assyrian word) Onyx is a form of quartz and many other stones have been wrongly labeled as onyx (a wrongly labeled stone would be a form of Calcite). Its predominant colours are black and white, though can range through all colours. Onyx was used in the second Dynasty in Egypt for making pottery items (a mix of, such as bowls) The purest source is in Brazil and it has a hardness rating of 7

Healing Ability: **Nervous system, hair, eyes, sleep disorders, heart, kidney, and reduces stress levels**

Magical Ability: **Attack enemies on a psychic level, attack enemies sexual energy, change habits, and reduce negative thoughts**

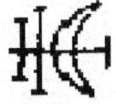

MOLDAVITE: Grail Stone – Grid of Czech Republic

The colour of Moldavite is green and is formed by the impact of a meteorite. Its purest source is from the Czech Republic, although there are four key sites around the world. It is regarded as having extra-terrestrial properties, certainly supernatural. This is a Grail Stone, able to enhance the alchemical transformation, and is twenty million years old. It is recognised that within a decade this Scared Grail Stone will no longer be available.

Healing Ability: Translates energy into reality within the physical existence, removes negative energies, regulates the heart, and is able to re-align the energies of existence

Magical Ability: Removes negative energies, regulates the internal mind, and awakens the spirit within.

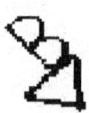

TEKTITE (WITH SANDSTONE): Hidden Knowledge – Grid of China

The colour of this form of Tektite is Black. It is formed by the impact of a meteorite. This particular form is located in China, although there are four key sites around the world. It is regarded as having extra-terrestrial properties. It is recognised that by most that this stone will bring knowledge to the beholder.

Healing Ability: Translates energy into reality within the physical existence, removes negative energies, and regulates the heart

Magical Ability: Removes negative energies, regulates the internal mind, and awakens the Hidden Knowledge.

CITRINE: Peace – Grid of Brazil

Citrine has a range colour of yellow to brown, yet transparent. Its name originated form the French word for lemon (citron). Its main source is Brazil and said that the holder will connect with spirit (with energies).

Healing Ability: Stimulates memory, calms depression, removal of toxins, assists digestion, liver, kidney, stabilises diabetes, and regulates the heart

Magical Ability: Enhances creativity, encourages happiness, reflects peace, protects when worn as a pendant

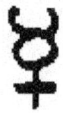

CALCITE: Success – Grid of New Mexico, America

Calcite contains particles of calcium. Its colour varies from white, cream, green, and even purple. It is known within the building industry, within paint as filler, and further used in optical instruments. Calcite has a harness rating of 3 and its pure source is found in New Mexico, America. The colour of Calcite varies from white, colourless, and yellow.

Healing Ability: Skin diseases, warts, ulcers, and the treating of general wounds, and stimulates the metabolism

Magical Ability: Stimulates ability, enhances trust, generates magical energies, enhances memory, and promotes success

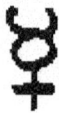

BLOODSTONE

Bloodstone is also known as 'Heliotrope', the colour of green with red spots or flecks (sometimes yellow flecks). It is a combination of green and red Jasper and said to represent the Sun setting upon the ocean. It is further associated with the crucifixion of Christ myth. Sources of Bloodstone can be located in Brazil, China, Australia and India. However the purest source is located in the United States of America. Bloodstone has a hardness rating of 7.

Healing Ability: Reduces confusion and anxiety, cleanses the blood (detoxifies the body); removes energy blocks, slows bleeding, and especially reduces nosebleeds. It is further used to aid the immune system by fighting infections. In ancient Egypt Bloodstone would be used in the treatment of tumours.

Magical Ability: Prolongs life, enhances wealth, overcomes enemies, and opens doors within the cycle of life. Enhances spells and assists to control negative spirits.

BLUE JOHN (FLUORITE)

The name Blue John comes from the French term 'bleu et jaune', meaning 'blue and yellow' due to its colour. Blue John is fluorite from Castleton, Derbyshire, in England. Its colour is purple through to blue, and has a harness rating of 4.

Healing Ability: Helps to ground excessive energy, assists energy blockages, respiratory conditions, arthritis, and skin conditions

Magical Ability: Focuses the mind, reveals truth, works with conscious minds, and reduces depression

MOSS AGATE

Moss Agate is also known as 'Mocha Stone', a white Stone with inclusions of green (the colour from chrome or iron metals). Usually formed in volcanic rocks, it is found in large volumes in America, but its purest source is located in Germany. It has a hardness rating of 7.

Healing Ability: Good for assisting women during pregnancy (reduces pain during delivery), develops strength, assists with self-expression and communication, a good stone for colds and influenza.

Magical Ability: An emotional healer, it assists with the truth, encourages honesty, increases the power of spells, and encourages friendship. A magical stone for wealth, happiness, and longevity

AMAZONITE

Amazonite is sometimes called 'Amazon Stone'. Its name was taken from the Amazon River where the majority were sourced. Sourced from Sweden, Germany and America. It purest source is located Madagascar, Africa. Amazonite is bright green in colour due to the level of lead within its composition. It does fracture easily, and has a hardness rating of 6.

Healing Ability: Used in the treatment of the nervous system and brain, Enhances understanding and creativity, inspires thought, balances energy, and stabilises communication

Magical Ability: Considered a Holy stone, it is said to bring success to the wearer. Used when communicating with the Spirits of the Dead (Gidim).

GARNET (PYROPE GARNET):

The name 'Garnet' comes from the Latin term 'Granatus', meaning grain. In particular, the form that is best used is 'Pyrope garnet', from the Latin 'Pyropos', meaning 'fire-eyed'. Its colour is black, through to deep red, though the transparency determines the use for Sacred Stones (i.e. gem stones). There are wide spectrums of colours, ranging from brown, black, green, yellow, orange, red, purple, and colourless. Interesting that Ancient Egyptian ritual tools and pendants were crafted from Pyrope garnet. *(For higher degrees and Sanctuary) Garnet is a family of minerals having similar physical and crystalline properties. They all have the same general chemical formula, $A_3B_2(SiO_4)_3$, where A can be calcium, magnesium, ferrous iron, or manganese, and B can be aluminum, ferric iron, or chromium, or in rare instances, titanium.*

Garnet is located in many places, including Greenland, Canada, Africa, and America; it is best sourced from Kazakhstan (Ex-Russian Empire), and has a hardness rating of 6.0 to 7.5.

Healing Ability: A stone of love and passion, it is said to enhance sexuality, intimacy, boost positive thoughts, and energy. . It is further considered to be good for the heart, lungs, arthritis, pancreas, varicose veins, toenails, testicles, and blood.

Magical Ability: Protects from negative energies and will reflect such energy back to the sender with immense strength. A magical healer, able to align the body's energy pattern and vibrate the tune of life. For the Magical Practitioner, Garnet is able to strengthen and enhance the ritual workings and Rites of Passage, with increased general strength, intensified power, cheers spirit and friendship convokes the spirits and power of fire, promotes courage, and protects the holder in travel and in war.

Garnet also symbolises the term **Alpha and Omega**, being from the phrase 'I am the alpha and the omega', an appellation of Enki (i.e. Jesus) in the Book of revelation (verses 1:8, 21:6, and 22:13) where it reads 'I am the Alpha and Omega,

AR: MULLEIN LEAF: Solar Spirit (Tasmania) - Ar – Sun – Life Giver – South – Grid of Poland - 20 – Orange – Dark Amber

The name of Amber was known as Ambre (Old English), Ambra (Latin), and Anbar Ambergris (Arabic). Although Amber is found in Norway, Denmark and England and has been washed to the coast. The purest form is found in Poland. It is said that the holder will feel happiness and has been used since 8000 B.C.E, though is not considered to be an anniversary gemstone.

Mullein leaf is native to Tasmania (an Australian Island)

Physical Use: Respiratory Tract Infections, digestive system, glandular swellings, and bronchial congestion (brewed as a tea with honey and boiling water), Placed in shoes to assist circulation, as a paste for inflammatory skin conditions (paste is made with olive oil)

Magical Use: Banishes Negativity, Defeats Enemies, Clarity and Insight, Life Giver, Good Luck, Attunes Magnetic Forces, Calms Aggression, and Stimulates Mental Focus. A key use in exorcism

LAHMU: APPLE LEAF / SEED: Watcher of the Plain (Russia) - Lahmu - Venus – Insight – East – Grid of Japan - 50 – Black - Obsidian

Obsidian is sourced from the magnetic grid of Japan. The colour of Obsidian is black, a natural glass formed by volcanic lava that cooled quickly. Other colours found in Obsidian are: brown, red, blue, grey, and green. Snowflake Obsidian is where there are bubbles or crystals in the stone. The Apple leaf/seed is native to Kazakhstan in Russia; the region was known as Alma-Ata, meaning 'the father of apples' and in today's world the city is named Almaty.

Physical Use: Realignment of Energy, Bones, Head, and Stimulates Brain Activity, colon cancer, prostate cancer, lung cancer, heart disease, weight loss, cholesterol.

Magical Use: Insight, Travel through the Plain(s), Raising Energy, and Energy Stability

ARATA: RASPBERRY LEAF: Watcher of the Plain (England) - Arata – The Earth – The Gift – West – Grid of South Africa - 40 – Brown – Tiger's Eye

Tiger's Eye was known as Cat's Eye, African Cat's Eye, and Crocidolite. The purest form is found in South Africa and is given in the 9th year of Handfastings. The Raspberry Leaf is native to England and considered the plant of future times

Physical Use: Make in a tea with honey and boiling water to calm pain, assist diabetes and cardiovascular health. Can further aid Asthma, Kidney, and High Blood Pressure. Make with a paste using olive oil for elasticity and inflammatory infections (i.e. Psoriasis)

Magical Use: Comforts the weak and sick, Focuses the Mind, Protection during Travel, and aid visualisation

ANUNNA: MANDRAKE ROOT: Watcher of the Plain - Anunna – Mars – Fertility, Initiative – South – Grid of Brazil - 3 – Red – Carnelian

Carnelian is also known as cornelian, from the Latin word meaning horn. The colour is from bright orange to reddish orange. Carnelian will be a deeper red dependant on the iron oxide. It is placed in the sun to change any tints to red, and has a hardness rating of 7. The purest form of Carnelian is found in Brazil. Mandrake Root is native to Southern Europe and is poisonous (Not to be consumed). The meaning of the name is that of the 'Love Plant' and sacred geometry applied to the numbers 6 and 16.

Physical Use: Assists conception and during pregnancy, Aids the Dying Process, Headaches, Nausea, Blood, Liver, Speech, and Infection

Magical Use: Hex Craft, Raising the Dead (The soul of the hanged man), Comforts to the weak or sick, enables courage, and empowers creativity

INANNA: WHITE WILLOW BARK: Watcher of the Plain (Iraq) - Inanna – Saturn – Sexual – East – Grid of Russia -15 – White – Clear Quartz

The purest form of Quartz is from Russia. It is also known as Krustallos, from the Greek word meaning ice. The colour has different names; the transparent quartz is a rock crystal, Brown quartz is known as Smokey quartz. There is a Rose quartz and even Amethyst. It is not considered to be an anniversary stone. Quartz has a hardness rating of 7. White Willow Bark is native to Europe and Asia, It is considered to be the essence of relieving pain and in particular, for use within reducing fever.

Physical Use: Ground into a powder to reduce fevers and calm pain. When made into a paste form (with the use of olive oil), it will sooth rheumatism. Also known use in treatment of nausea, infection, and sexual problems, and lethargy

Magical Use: In a pure state for healing and love spells. When in a powder form it is best applied to conjurations. May further be used for visions of the future, raising power, and cleansing space

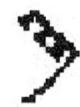

EA: HOLLY LEAF: Watcher of the Plain (America) - Ea – Neptune – Communication – South – Grid of Egypt -12 – Blue – Blue Lace Agate

The purest form of Agate is found in Egypt. The holly leaf is native to America. The holly leaf should be used with caution and in particular, the berries are poisonous. Note that 20 berries constitute a lethal dose. Before the Yule tree was born Craft would hang a large ball of evergreen and holly within the home at Yule. From the ball would be draped red, white, and black ribbon and paper roses, apples, and oranges.

Physical Use: Make into a paste with olive oil to reduce wrinkles, calm arthritis, and cleanse facial tissue. Add the paste to oil within a burner in the home to reveal the truth of suspicion.

Magical Use: Place above a door to prevent enemies from entering and to encourage useful spirits to enter. Further used with Spell Craft for raising energy and for communication across the five plains. Holly leaves under a pillow will enhance travel within dreams.

NABU: LILY LEAF: The Inner Sanctum (China) - Nabu – Mercury – Protection – Hidden East – Grid of Germany - 60 – Red (and sometimes Orange) – Jasper

The name Jasper was known as Iaspis (Greek) and the purest form is found in Germany. The colour of Jasper is red, brown, green, greyish-blue, and yellow. Often jasper is multi-colour and has a hardness rating of 7. Lily leaf is known as the plant of summer and abundance, it is one of the three holy flowers, a symbol of purity and long associated with love and with death.

Physical Use: Hold the Lily Leaf upon your person to promote strength and good luck. Grind into a powder to cure depression and create harmony within the home. Make a paste using olive oil and use as a facial moisturiser, or burn within the bedroom to promote sleep.

Magical Use: Enables sight of the Gidim and enhances sexual desires within males. Further used within Hex Craft to harm those who attack.

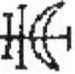

<u>ANU: BURDOCK ROOT:</u> **Watcher of the Plain (North America) - Anu – Uranus – Existence – West – Grid of America - 13 – Black (and sometimes Blue) - Hematite**

The name Hematite is also known as Haematite, from the haem name for blood (Greek). In ancient times Hematite objects were made and placed in tombs. The colour of Hematite has the appearance of silvery metal, but when ground turns to a red powder as if it were bleeding. It has a hardness rating of 6.5. Burdock root is long and fleshy with the outer skin being grey and brown and white inside. The root can be eaten as a root vegetable and is often shredded with carrots. As a root vegetable, it is often died orange to image the carrot for consumer favour.

Physical Use: A mild laxative and diuretic, use as an antibiotic, and purification of blood. As a paste (with olive oil) it is used for the treatment of boils, abscesses, Psoriasis, and Eczema. Further used for Venereal Disease, and known to strengthen the body.

Magical Use: High increase to psychic powers, inspires inner life, enables creation of individual sphere of protection

NAMMU: SAGE: *Higher Intelligence (Mexico) - Nammu – Universal – Creation – Hidden Grid of Afghanistan - 9 – Yellow – Lapis Lazuli*

The colour of Lapis Lazuli is shades of blue, some with speckled of veining white (Calcite) or yellow (Pyrite). It buried with the dead to guide them towards the L.i.g.h.t. It is given in the 7th and 9th year of Handfastings. Sage is a small evergreen shrub with silver to grey leaves. The name derives from the Latin name 'Salvia' meaning 'to heal'.

Physical Use: Internally in the management of Alzheimer's disease, use as an antibiotic and antifungal. Further calms anxiety and liver complaints. Reduces negative emotions, and soothes throat pain. *Do not use if pregnant or you have epilepsy*

Magical Use: Used within Purification Rites and immortality spells. Will further protect against those who may attack. Sage is able to focus energy and reflect any negative magic used back to the creator. Offerings of Sage must be made to the black flame at Mabon and at Yule.

RA.UBAN: AGRIMONY: The Unknown Master (Africa) - With One – Spiritual Connection – Hidden Site of England - 5 – Black – Serpentine – The Black Sun

The name Serpentine was named due to its colour and marking similar to that of a snake. It has a direct connection to all that is spiritual both on the plain and in time itself, being of purpose in time and travel. The name Agrimony is from the Greek name 'Argemone' which mean to be healing to the eyes. It is a deep green plant with soft hairs.

Physical Use: Place within a cloth bag under the pillow to cure insomnia. As a paste (mixed with olive oil) it is used in the treatment of acne. Mixed with water it may be used as a mouthwash to relieve inflamed gums and sore throats. Absorbs Negative Emotions, Reflects Negative patterns in the biochemistry, and is able to regulate the hypothalamus.

Magical Use: Blocks and reflects negative Spells, able to raise the seal of 333, and further used for protection seals during Sacred Rites.

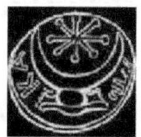

SHUPA: KELP: The Inner Sanctum (California, America) - Shupa – Pluto – Guardian – West – Grid of Spain Church of St. Mary – Guadalajara – Spain - 60 – Black - Aragonite

Aragonite is best sourced from Aragon in Spain (Where its name was given), it may be further sourced from Morocco, France, Sicily, England (Cumbria), United States, and Mexico. It is said that the holder will obtain future insight. Kelp is a large seaweed belonging to the brown algae family. Kelp grows in underwater forests and is suited to shallow, clear oceans with temperatures below 20⊕c. It is known for its fast growing rate.

Physical Use: Assists the thyroid gland by regulating the body's metabolic rate. Further used in a paste form for muscle spasms and as a face wash for physical perfection.

Magical Use: Increased psychic powers, disciplines the mind. Kelp is particularly prominent in sea and wind spells.

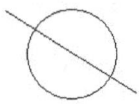

ANSHAR: HAWTHORN: Watcher of the Plain (Northwest Africa) - Anshar – Moon – Damuzi Existence – North – Grid of America Old Faithful Geyser, Calistoga – California – America - 30 – Silver - Howlite

Howlite can be green, white, or blue. A calming stone and if placed on the 'inner mind' or rather the third eye can assist with travelling outside the body to past, present, and the future. The Hawthorn is native to northwest Africa, and particular attention should be drawn to the legend of the staff on the hill in Glastonbury, England. It should further be noted that this legend began in 37 CE, and thus considered a new concept. The flowers of the Hawthorn are used at the Beltane Ritual.

Physical Use: Used in the treatment of heart and circulatory problems. As a tea it will reduce stress, strengthen bones and teeth, and purify the blood.

Magical Use: Marks the entrance to the Plain(s), brings good luck and prosperity to the land where it is planted. Worn as a talisman for psychic protection. The magical properties will cleanse the Aura.

KISHAR: LAVENDER: The Inner Sanctum (India) - Kishar – Jupiter – Strength – North – Grid of America Tequiquiapan Volcanic Springs – Mexico -60 – Jupiter - Azurite
Also found in Otavi, Namibia. The name for Azurite originates from a Persian term, meaning 'blue'. Lavender is native to India with a multitude of purposes from dried flower arrangements through to sachets for stored clothes to maintain a fresh fragrance.

Physical Use: used as an antiseptic for walls and floors, applied to the temples for relief of headaches, or burn as incense in the bedroom to aid sleep. Place around the home to promote peace and harmony, or carry upon your person for strength. Further assists arthritis in a paste form. *Do not use if pregnant or breastfeeding*

Magical Use: Activates expansion of consciousness, stimulates psychic abilities, clearer meditation, enhances inspiration, and assists with mental control. Further enhances sexual desire in males.

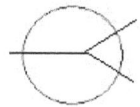

NABU: MARJORAM: The Inner Sanctum - Nabu – Mercury – Protection – Hidden East – Grid of Germany -60 – Red (and sometimes Orange) - Jasper

Marjoram is an under shrub with a sweet citrus flavour. A member of the mint family, and is often confused with the Greek Oregano. Marjoram grows thirty to sixty centimetres tall and has slightly hairy ovate leaves.

Physical Use: Frequently used for flavouring meat, poultry, fish, and stews. Marjoram may be burnt and used as an air freshener. Mix into a paste (with olive oil) to ease spasms, stimulate circulation, and to reduce ageing of the skin.

Magical Use: Enables love, purification, happiness, and wealth. Combine Marjoram with mint and rosemary to sprinkle in an area as a form of protection.

NABU: MARSHMALLOW LEAVES: The Inner Sanctum - Nabu – Mercury – Protection – Hidden East – Grid of Germany - 60 – Red (and sometimes Orange) - Jasper

Marshmallow is a member of the hollyhock family. In times past the gum was extracted from the root and processed into sugars as a sweetener for candy.

Physical Use: Marshmallow has anti-infective properties. Make into a teas then soak in a non-adhesive material for eye infections and boils. Inhale in steam baths to ease congestion and coughing. Mix into a paste (with olive oil) to soothe chapped skin, insect bites, or use as a moisturiser. Marshmallow is particularly good for leg ulcers.

Magical Use: Carry in a sachet for protection. Marshmallow enables psychic powers during rituals and especially good for visualisations.

LAHMU: EUCALYPTUS: Watcher of the Plain -
Lahmu - Venus – Insight – East – Grid
of Japan - 50 – Black - Obsidian

Eucalyptus is native to Australia and ranges in height from ten to sixty metres tall. The leaves are evergreen.

Physical Use: Can be used as a disinfectant, but poisonous in large amounts. Mix into a paste (with olive oil) for healing insect bites, cuts, headaches, and colds.

Magical Use: Enables love, purification, stimulates the creation of energy. May be used in Blessing Rites, but more useful within Hex Craft.

LAHMU: MUGWORT: Watcher of the Plain - Lahmu - Venus – Insight – East – Grid of Japan -- 50 – Black – Obsidian. For higher degrees

Mugwort is native to North Africa and is found in wet places and busy areas. It has grooved stems that grow one to two metres tall. It is essential to note that Mugwort is a different species of 'Wormwood'. The leaves are dark green underneath. ***Caution** High doses are poisonous. Avoid if pregnant*

Physical Use: Can be used as a bath additive for gout and is good for stimulating the nervous system. Mix Mugwort into a paste (with olive oil) for tired muscles and rheumatism.

Magical Use: Enables strength, psychic powers, protection, dream travelling, and general healing. Place Mugwort in a sachet under a pillow to aid travelling the plains. When it is burnt it will aid exorcism.

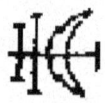

KISHAR: HONEYSUCKLE: The Inner Sanctum - Kishar – Jupiter – Strength – North – Grid of America (Stone: Tequiquiapan Volcanic Springs – Mexico) - 60 – Jupiter - Azurite

Honeysuckle is native to China and is further known as 'Woodbine'. The Honeysuckle leaves are one to ten centimetres long, and the herb is able to climb up to ten metres tall.

Caution should not be used by the weak or the elderly

Physical Use: Honeysuckle has antibacterial and anti-inflammatory properties and is the ideal herb for removing toxins. Make into a paste (with olive oil) to cure ulcers, fever,

influenza, and skin conditions. Add to a bath for re-energising. It will assist the lungs, stomach, and intestines when burnt within a room.

Magical Use: Enables prosperity and assists with the use of the spirit board (channel board). Particularly useful for binding lovers, though caution should be the key word for this purpose. Apply to the forehead as a light oil to enhance psychic powers.

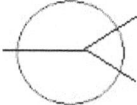

ANSHAR: CAMPHOR: Watcher of the Plain - Anshar – Moon – Damuzi Existence – North – Grid of America - Old Faithful Geyser, Calistoga – California – America - 30 – Silver - Howlite

Camphor is collected from the evergreen tree 'Camphor Laurel' and native to Taiwan. Camphor is a transparent solid with an aromatic odour.

Caution this herb is poisonous in high doses

Physical Use: Used for flavouring sweets and in small doses for general cooking. Further used in the making of embalming fluid, or as a scent. Make into a paste (with olive oil) and apply to the skin as a mild anaesthetic. It is an anti-itch agent, and is able to reduce congestion. Reduces chapped or rough skin, and particularly good for the feet.

Magical Use: Enhances sexual desires and assists in love. When camphor is burnt it is a symbol of the consciousness. It is best used within ritual for raising and controlling spirits.

ANUNNA: WORMWOOD: Watcher of the Plain - Anunna – Mars – Fertility, Initiative – South – Grid of Brazil - 3 – Red – Carnelian

Wormwood is a shrub which is native to North Africa. It has grey to white stems that are covered in fine silk hairs. Wormwood grows between thirty to ninety centimetres tall.

Caution Can be addictive. May cause nausea, vomiting and insomnia; people with Epilepsy should avoid

Physical Use: Wormwood has strong antifungal and antibacterial properties. It is best used for the treatment of hepatitis, fever, liver, gallbladder, and general infections. When burnt in a room it will help to boost the immune system, and aid the clearing of toxins. Make into a paste (with olive oil) for arthritis, skin conditions, insect bites, and insect stings.

Magical Use: Assists in communication when used with the Spirit Board (Channel Board), empowers protection, increases psychic powers, and regulates the body's energy patterns. Wormwood is the ideal herb for Samhain.

AR: ROSEMARY: The Solar Spirit of Time - Ar – The Sun – Life Giver – South – Grid of Poland - 20 – Orange – Dark Amber

Rosemary is a member of the mint family, growing up to one and a half metres tall. Rosemary derives from the Latin term 'rosmarinus' meaning 'dew of the sea'. Its leaves are evergreen and needle-like.

Physical Use: Assists the nervous system. Make into a paste (with olive oil) then add to water for pre-ritual cleansing. Rosemary is used as a representation of union when used within Handfasting Ceremonies, being the suitable replacement of confetti. Is appropriate to use within a Funeral Rite, where onlookers cast the rosemary to the grave.

Magical Use: Aids intellectual achievements, assists purification, protection, and love. Use rosemary within the Last Rites Service.

AR: FRANKINCENSE: The Solar Spirit of Time
- Ar – The Sun – Life Giver – South – Grid of Poland - 20 – Orange – Dark Amber

Frankincense is obtained from the Bosarellia tree by slashing the bark to allow the resins to seep out, and then harden. It is best sourced from Somalia in East Africa.

Physical Use: Used by the Egyptians to make black eyeliner, in modern times Frankincense is best used as a deodoriser. Make into a paste (with olive oil) to re-energise areas of the body.

Magical Use: Assists purification, protection, exorcism, and love. Frankincense is mixed with olive oil and black salt when used in Naming Ceremonies.

AR: MURGH (MYRRH): The Solar Spirit of Time - Ar – The Sun – Life Giver – South – Grid of Poland - 20 – Orange – Dark Amber

Murgh in modern times is spelt 'Myrrh'. It is native to Somalia, East Africa and is dried sap from the 'Commiphora Myrrha'. Murgh was introduced to the English language from the ancient Greeks, with its smoke being heavy and bitter in the air.

Physical Use: Used in mixtures of incense. Mix into a paste (with olive oil) to assist circulation, arthritis, or use as a facial moisturiser. When made into a mouth wash (just add water to the paste) it can be used to gargle with to reduce gum disease.

Magical Use: Used within Funeral Rites to cleanse the soul, and at Yule to re-start the cycles of the Earth.

OLIVE LEAF / OIL:

Olive Leaf is the leaf from an olive tree. Ancient Egyptians used the Olive Lead for medicinal use. It is an antioxidant, therefore assisting the removal of free radical from the body.

Physical Use: Antioxidant (reduce free radicals), assists in the treatment of the Liver, Tumours, and Cancer

Magical Use: Assists with focusing the mind, opening the soul, raising energy, manifestations, and travel the spheres of time

SULPHUR BRIMSTONE:

Sulphur (oftentimes referred to as Brimstone) is an essential element of life, having 'amino acids', and is often referred to a smelling like the dwelling of the modern Christian concept of 'hell', this is far removed – In fact, this Sacred powder is used to awaken the senses and aid communication with the Goddess herself. Largely use in fertilizers, matches, and gunpowder; a substance that should be handled with care and respect. Locations of Sulphur can be found in Wales, America, Afghanistan, Iran, China, Japan, Russia, Australia, and New Zealand. The best source is from England (in particular; Wadebridge, Cornwall). *Should be handled in small portions, and with care*

Physical Use: Can help to remove negative thoughts and feelings, and is further consider to aid wellbeing. One of the components used to aid skin conditions and muscle aches.

Magical Use: Able to align the body's energy fields, and bring. When used within ritual, will assist in cleansing space to which you wish to work.

Grail Castle: Associated with Tourmaline and the Sword of Truth, the Planet of Venus and the Goddess within Mary Magdalene. (Amulug)

SOLOMON'S SEAL:

Solomon's seal is best sourced from North America, Asia, and Europe. It is typically 'woodland perennial'. It is similar to 'Lily of the Valley'.

Physical Use: Increases concentration, calms inflammation, and is good for assisting concentration. Made into a paste, this Sacred Herb can assist cuts, bruises, insect bites, general irritation, and inflammation

Magical Use: Will bring Wisdom, Knowledge, Good Fortune, and Positive Dreams (Great for reducing nightmares).

Grail Castle: Associated with Smokey Quartz and the Stone of Magnesite, the Planet of Mars and represents the within 'the internal thoughts, feelings, and soul' of the individual.

SALT PETRE: (Potassium Nitrate)

Saltpetre is also known as 'Salt Petre', form Latin, meaning; Stone Salt. Its chemical name is 'Potassium Nitrate', and has been used as an ingredient of fertilizer, smoke bombs, and gunpowder. *Should be handled in small portions, and with care*

Physical Use: When made into a paste with Olive Oil, it can help to alleviate the pain of angina and muscle spasms. Carefully crush a charcoal disc, sulphur (Brimstone), and Salt Petre, then add ash created from burnt wood only – Then add to an outside open fire during Fire Spirit Rituals.

Magical Use: Absorbs psychic energy – BUT, be careful – Salt Petre will absorb good and bad energies, so if used by the inexperienced, could restrict the magical practices of the user and others.

Grail Castle: Associated with Onyx and the Chalice of Existence, the Planet of Jupiter and represents the Son of the Holy 'Jul' (Nabu).

BELLADONNA: (Deadly Nightshade)

Belladonna is also known as 'Deadly Nightshade' for the very reason of being extremely toxic. It is known as having the properties to be hallucinogenic. Its name comes from Italy where women used to use Deadly Nightshade to enlarge the pupils of their eyes; hence the meaning of 'Belladonna' to be a 'Beautiful Woman'. *Should be handled in small portions, and with care*

Physical Use: Calms Pain, Assists sleep disorders and is added (in very small doses) to Olive Oil and Marshmallow Leaf for paste for muscular pain

Magical Use: Aids Visualisation and Dream Travel, aids the crossing during Funeral Rites. Belladonna Berries are especially good (in very small doses) as an ingredient for 'flying oils'

Grail Castle: Associated with Moldavite and the Wand of Direction, the Planet of Mercury and represents the Goat 'Durah' of the future.

MERCURY: Star – Connection between High and Low (Marshmallow)

A heavy, silvery metal, mercury is one of five metals that are liquid at or near room temperature and pressure. Mercury was known to the ancient Chinese and was transmutation of impure metals into gold. It is a rare element in the Earth's crust. However, it is important to recognise that as previously instructed, substitute with the ingredient Marshmallow leaf. Marshmallow is a member of the hollyhock family. In times past the gum was extracted from the root and processed into sugars as a sweetener for candy.

Physical Use: Marshmallow has anti-infective properties. Make into a teas then soak in a non-adhesive material for eye infections and boils. Inhale in steam baths to ease congestion and coughing. Mix into a paste (with olive oil) to soothe chapped skin, insect bites, or use as a moisturiser. Marshmallow is particularly good for leg ulcers.

Magical Use: Carry in a sachet for protection. Marshmallow enables psychic powers during rituals and especially good for visualisations.

Mercury

'*A drink or two from the hunter's source will surely make things right*'

'*Such creatures were for food and slavery*'

HEALING WITH SACRED STONES:
Introduction to the first sequence of stones

THE CHANNEL BOARD is the focus of this solar systems energy, or rather the magnetic forces contained within. We focus on the magnetic forces, as it is the foundation of positive and negative existence. By tuning in to the magnetic frequencies of the solar system, we are empowered to realise the Gifts from within. The sun magic (Solomon Magic) is of such force and direction; it is the principles of the solar system and true to the positive and negative frequencies that surround the mundane world.

The Channel Board (shown below) can be made of wood, (round breadboards and cork placemats are a very good size) or simply drawn on paper or card, sewn or drawn on to cloth, pyrographed into wood or inscribed upon the ground in the sequence as shown below:

Also known as the **Samna Emua** (Eighth Force)

(Having eight sacred stones aligned upon the board)

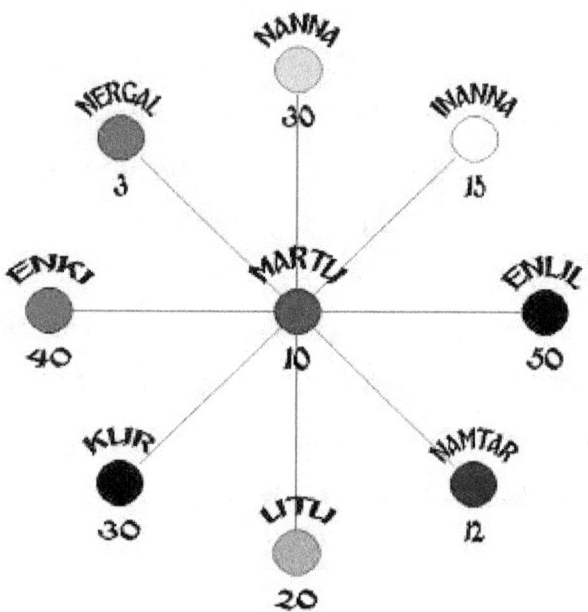

List of Stones needed and their placement upon the Channel Board

OBSIDIAN FOR KUR IN THE SOUTH-WEST – BLACK – MERCURY

The 13th House is Kur and of Mercury, the Guardian and protector of the boundary between the plains of Earth and the crossing to the spheres. His strength is of logic, intellect, and travel. Associated with communication, Kur is the decision maker on whether you will open the spheres to communicate with Deity. He is placed at the South-West quadrant as the balance of the Sun and Earth. Kur's planet of Mercury has a diameter of 4,888 KM and is 57,910,000 KM from the Sun and is the closest planet. The atmosphere is constantly refreshed by solar winds and the planet revolves around the sun in 88 days. Three times each Earth year, Mercury looks like it is retrograde for a three-week period. This means it looks like it is going backwards.

JASPER FOR RESHEPH IN THE EAST – RED – MARS

The 12th House is Resheph and of Mars, the hidden Deity of the East and that of plague and war. Resheph is called by Craft who have achieved the Elect Degree and above. His strength is of aggression, initiative, and power. Resheph's planet of Mars has a diameter of 6,794 KM and is 227,940,000 KM from the Sun. Early in history Mars was similar to Earth, having carbon dioxide. However, lacking plate tectonics it is unable to recycle and by this, unable to sustain a greenhouse effect.

FIRE OPAL FOR ISHKUR IN THE NORTH – ORANGE – JUPITER

The 11th House is Ishkur and of Jupiter, the hidden deity of the North and that of storms. Ishkur is called by Craft who have achieved the Elect Degree and above. His strength is of generosity and optimism. Ishkur's planet of Jupiter has a diameter of 142,984 KM and is 778,330,000 KM from the Sun. Jupiter orbits the Sun every 12 Earth years.

MOON STONE FOR NANNA IN THE NORTH – SILVER – MOON

The 10th House is Nanna and of Moon, a very old Deity. His strength is of parenthood and to nurture. Nanna's planet of Moon has a diameter of 3,476 KM and is 384,400 KM from Earth. Moon orbits Earth once every Earth month. As the Moon orbits, the angle of the Moon, Earth, and the Sun changes and we see this as the cycle of the moon phases.

HEMATITE FOR ERESHKIGAL IN THE WEST – BLACK – PLUTO

The 9th House is Ereshkigal and Pluto, the Destroyer and holder of the underworld. Ereshkigal is called by Craft who have achieved the Elect Degree and above. Her strength is of generosity and optimism and holds the secrets of the universe. She represents both fear and desire. Ereshkigal's planet Pluto has a diameter of 2,274 KM and is 5,913,520,000 KM from the Sun.

Pluto's orbit takes it closer to the Sun than Neptune. Pluto rotates in the opposite direction from most of the other planets.

CARNELIAN FOR NERGAL IN THE NORTH-WEST – RED – MARS

The 8th House is Nergal and shares the holding of the underworld with Ereshkigal. His strength is of plague and war. Nergal's planet Mars has a diameter of 6,794 KM and is 227,940,000 KM from the Sun. Early in history Mars was similar to Earth, having carbon dioxide. However, lacking plate tectonics it is unable to recycle and by this, unable to sustain a greenhouse effect.

AMETHYST FOR MARTU IN THE CORTEX – PURPLE – NIBIRU

The 7th House is Martu, the all seeing and all knowing. It is the place to travel the stars. Martu is called by Craft who have achieved the Elect Degree and above. The strength of Martu is that of travel and time. Martu's planet Nibiru has a diameter 146,143 KM and orbits the System every 3,600 Earth years.

BLUE LACE AGATE FOR NAMTAR IN THE SOUTH-EAST – BLUE – NEPTUNE

The 6th House is Namtar, the Messenger of Deity. His strength is of vengeance and disease. He represents communication and justice of all. Namtar governs illusions and spirituality, to be enlightened and is able to confuse and provide cosmic perspective at the same time. Namtar's planet Neptune has a diameter of 49,532 KM and is 4,504,000,000 KM from the Sun. Neptune is of ice and rock with a core or rock the size of Earth.

HEMATITE FOR NINLIL IN THE SOUTH – BLACK

The 5th House is Ninlil, the shape-shifter who often transforms into the owl, or a female human with wings. Her strength is invention and revolution. Ninlil is called by Craft who have achieved the Elect Degree and above.

Ninlil's planet of Uranus has a diameter of 51,118 KM and is 2,870,990,000 KM from the Sun. Uranus is of ice and rock with a rock core. It is of Hydrogen, Helium, and Methane.

AMBER FOR UTU IN THE SOUTH – ORANGE-SUN

The 4th House is Utu, the giver of life. His strength is of clarity and insight, being used well in future casting. He represents the negative and positive aspects of life, being balance and chaos at the same time. Utu's planet the Sun is 4.5 billion years old, and will continue for another 5 billion years. It has a diameter of 1,390,000 KM and contains hydrogen within its core

QUARTZ FOR INANNA IN THE NORTH-EAST – WHITE – SATURN

The 3rd House is Inanna the healer and of rebirth, the negative aspects confirm the warrior. If she appears in purest white she has manifested to assist. However, if she manifests and is wearing armour, then she is to do battle. Be certain of the binding spells if armour is raised as you will need to tame this wild entity. Inanna's planet Saturn has a diameter of 120,536 KM and is 1,429,400,000 KM from the Sun. Saturn is of hydrogen, helium, water, methane, ammonia, and rock. Saturn's day is 10 hours, 39 minutes long. It takes 29.5 Earth years to revolve about the Sun.

TIGER EYE FOR ENKI IN THE WEST – BROWN – EARTH

The 2nd House is Enki, the controller of all things natural on the plain. She is of nature's design, and nature's design is of her. Her strength is of the life-giver and the gift of nature's wisdom.

Enki's planet Earth has a diameter of 12,756.3 KM and is 149,600,000 KM from the Sun. Earth's chemical composition is of Iron, Oxygen, Silicon, Magnesium, Nickel, Sulphur, and Titanium.

OBSIDIAN FOR ENLIL IN THE EAST – BLACK – VENUS

The 1st House is Enlil, the Controller of air, space, and time. He is close to An and Nammu and is the mark of our race from beyond the stars. His strength in true form is to grant love and desire. Enlil's planet Venus has a diameter of 12,103.6 KM and is 108,200,000 KM from the Sun. The atmosphere of Venus is mainly carbon dioxide. For each day on Venus, 243 Earth days occur. This is due to Venus having a slow rotational motion and being retrograde (rotational motion clockwise).

However, it is important to take on board the caution within this lecture and usage of the board; that is the caution of 'cause and affect'. It is the key concern of each Practitioner of the Craft; for example, if we were to draw the force of Nergal or Namtar into our ritual to cause a disturbance within an individual's life cycle, this may have an adverse affect either on the Practitioner himself or herself, or even an innocent party. The Practitioner's understanding of the Channel Board is essential as he or she may need to harmonise their affect, or even strengthen their affect caused within a ritual. The Channel Board contains the Hidden Mysteries and more importantly the 'Key to the Mystery' within the Knights Templar teachings. It not only looks and feels powerful it is powerful. Each direction on the Board has been set to an exact measurement, precise magnetic force tuning, and identifies the planetary sequence of alignments. The Deity's magnetic force is associated with the magnetic map of the Earth and can be best displayed as a guide in the following:

SUMMARY:

8 Channel Stones - 3 Hidden Stones – 2 Universal Stones

AMBER (C) Healing Ability: Eyes, Lungs, Throat, Digestive System, and Glandular Swellings
Magical Ability: Clarity and Insight, Life Giver, Good Luck, Longevity, Attunes Magnetic Forces, Calms Aggression, and Stimulates Mental Focus

OBSIDIAN (C) Healing Ability: Realignment of Energy, Bones, Head, and Stimulates Brain Activity
Magical Ability: Insight, Underworld Travel, and Energy Stability

TIGER'S EYE (C) Healing Ability: Asthma, Kidney, Heart Disease, Psoriasis, and High Blood Pressure
Magical Ability: Provides comfort to the weak and sick, Focuses the Mind, and Protection during Travel

MOONSTONE (C) Healing ability: Aligns vertebrae, Assists Digestion, Fertility, and Balances Emotion

Magical Ability: Protection, Good Fortune, and Arouses Passion

CARNELIAN (C) Healing Ability: Headaches, Nausea, Blood, Liver, Speech, and Infection

Magical Ability: Provides comfort to the weak or sick, enables courage, to cause sudden noise or disturbance. Also for Good Luck and will empower creativity

CLEAR QUARTZ (C) Healing Ability: Nausea, Infection, and sexual problems, Lethargy

Magical Ability: Visions of Future, Raising Power, and Cleansing Space

BLUE LACE AGATE (C) Healing Ability: Damaged Skin, Reawakens cell tissue, Rash, General Skin Infection, Soothes Discomfort, Arthritis, Bones, Pancreas, Blood Sugar Balance, Bites, and Stings

Magical Ability: Communication, Raising Power, to defeat enemies, and Protection during travels

AMETHYST (C) Healing Ability: Psychic Ability, Brain Activity, Strengthens immunity, purifies the blood, Headaches, and Blood Sugars
Magical Ability: Aids Drunkenness (either positive of negative), Love Charms, Protection against Theft, Calms Sleep, Enables Travel in Dream State, Insight to Solve Problems, Raise Energy, Charge Soul and Body, and enhances Spirituality

FIRE OPAL (H) Healing Ability: Heart, Feet, Hands, Circulation, and Muscular
Magical Ability: Attunes to Higher Plains, Heightens Awareness, used during the Crowning Ceremony

JASPER (H) Healing Ability: Stomach, gynaecological problems, Depression,
Magical Ability: Brings Joy and drives away those who attack

HEMATITE (H) Healing Ability: Hysteria, Bladder, Venereal Disease, and Strengthens Body, venereal diseases

Magical Ability: General Healing, resistance to life's stress, inspires inner life, keeps inward peace

LAPIS LAZULI (U) Healing Ability: Increase Abilities, Fever, Negative Emotions, and Throat Pain

Magical Ability: Clarity, Calm, Focusing Energy, Enhances Spirituality, and Raising Power

CITRINE (U) Ability: This stone is sealed within a Fire Opal Seal and used as if it were Amethyst. Its healing abilities are absorbed in the same way as Amethyst; practitioners of a 19th Degree (Grand Pontiff), or lower Degree should not attempt to use it

'Expectations are an illusion – Allow one's mind to open'

CLEANSING OF SACRED STONES BEFORE OR AFTER USE:

For all water cleansing use the Cleansing Chant below and be sure to hold your left hand straight out using a Widdershins motion (anti-clockwise) commence the Chant over the chalice of water, whilst repeating the cleansing chant. Finish with a swift motion to the left.

Uru Annu Da A Dimmu Antam Keezh Annu Arazu
Be Gi Ma Dag Wur Damu Ma Bar Bana Gan-Kan-Kha
Ina Ara Ma Ina Ina Zagduku

Guard this Gift I order the Universe
Under this Prayer to be night and day
Wisdom Child and seat of wisdom
Exorcise this Vessel in time and in the dark threshold

Dip stones or other working tools into the water to cleanse; also to be used for cleansing hands prior to working.

USE OF SACRED STONES FOR HEALING

You will need the Channel Board and above listed Sacred Stones

Now that you have a basic understanding of the stones and their purpose, we can start with our Channel Board for use within our practice. Have all stones aligned on the Channel Board as instructed above and hold the Lapis Lazuli tight in your left palm. Raise your hand (Knuckles upwards) over the Channel Board and focus on the energy contained within. Gently start a Widdershins motion (anti-clockwise) around the board. The speed of the motion is for you to decide, but ensure that all energy attunes to you appropriately. You will know when the stones are ready. Now continue with the Widdershins motion and say this Mystic Chant:

E-gish-shir-gal e-gish-shir-gal lu annu bi ma lalartu eri

(House of great light) (house of great light) (let this divide) (and phantom bind)

Now either permit the Recipient to choose, or you may choose the two stones for use in the treatment **One Stone is chosen for its MAGICAL ABILITY, and the other stone for its HEALING ABILITY** Now place both Chosen stones into the chalice of water and with your LEFT hand flat, you may perform the '*Script of Namtar*', once again widdershins around the chalice:

Resheph kur dingar e ina utu, nanna, ma adar su'ati annu piriq ina azag annu tisa bi er e gallas mamman aga azag bur annu aka annu wur eri

(Resheph underworld god) (raise the sun, moon and star) (that this the bearer of the magic) (from the shining bright) (this ninth command to go raise demons) (whoever crowns the shining bright) (hear this divine command) (this wisdom bind)

The recipient now takes the two sacred chosen stones from the chalice and grasps them in their hands as detailed:

The **Magical** ability to be placed in the recipient's **Left** hand.
The **Healing** ability to be placed in the recipient's **Right** hand.

The recipient will now lie down on their back, holding the chosen stones in the appropriate hands, then release the stones to naturally fall either in front of the finger tips, or below each palm, whilst lying down.

Now go to the prepared chalice of water and cleanse you hands in the water, when you feel thoroughly cleansed and charged, start at the top of the recipient's head and slowly work around the body.

Your hands must not touch the recipient, but flow over the body for as long as you feel is required – you are the only judge in this domain – it is best that your hands flow over the recipients body at about 4 – 10 centimetres away.

Now ask the recipient to hand you the sacred stones, dip them quickly into the chalice of water and place directly back onto the channel board. Once again with the left hand and straightened out, move your hand deosil (clockwise) around the channel board, then quickly off the board to seal the energies.

You have now completed the first stage of psychic healing with stones.

You may practice the 'charging' of the channel board as many times as you wish, always finishing by 'sealing' the board as instructed. Practice makes perfect and in time you will discover and truly 'feel' for yourself how the aligned stones work together. Please practice thoroughly each section before moving on to the next.

'It is only the man who shows gratitude that will truly be enlightened'

SERPENTINE, OBSIDIAN, ARAGONITE AND HOWLITE

SERPENTINE:

As instructed above, the Samnu Emua or Eighth Force is used for one purpose, of aligning the healing and magical abilities of the Practitioner to the Recipient. However, this is merely one element of this working tool. We must venture further into the aspect of protection for the Practitioner and the use of the Samnu Emua for ritual work.

The stone we are now working with is the stone of work, the Serpentine or Sinser, to be kept and held for as long as you have strength to perform; its purity will work with you:

This stone has the name Serpentine due to its markings and colour represented by the snake. It is sourced from South Africa, Italy, China, New Zealand, America, England, and Italy. Although Serpentine is commonly known as a healing stone, its use suits the Practitioner to have on their person so to absorb, reflect, and destroy the negative physical and magical forces that yearn to harm the Practitioner.

This stone has a unique setting when performing any form of magical curse to another. It should therefore, not be used by a Practitioner until first being fully confident and knowledgeable with the Channel Board healings. Serpentine is used against others for blocking magical levels, imbalance on a physical level, to halt progression of the design, and most importantly, to halt dreams and desires of another.

It is a stone that should not be used lightly and consider your own level of morality before using the stone in this way. Let us now perform the script of Namtar, so to charge this stone to you as the holder, making you one with the stone:

THE SCRIPT OF NAMTAR:

(To charge the stone so the Practitioner becomes the holder: Performed widdershins with Serpentine in the left hand, grasped with knuckles upward; hand travelling widdershins around the SAMNU EMUA - Eighth Force – Once the script has been performed, take the hand off the board, to the left, in a sharp motion)

Gi Be Dag Ma Dara Be Ar E Ina Utu, Nanna, Ma Adar Su'ati Annu Piriq Ina Azag Annu Bi Be Sinser Er E Gallas Mamman Aga Azag Bur Annu Aka Annu Wur Eri

Night to be Day and Dark to be Light Raise the sun, moon and star That this the bearer of the magic From the shining bright This command to be twelve to go raise demons Whoever crowns the shining bright hear this divine command This wisdom bind

Now that the Serpentine is charged to you, if you wish to loan your stone to another to absorb their negativity, ensure that upon its return, you cleanse the stone as you were taught above, using the cleansed water.

If you wish to perform the following ritual against another, then you will be required to charge the stone for the purpose on each occasion:

SERPENTINE AGAINST ANOTHER:

You will need a candle, an offering bowl or dish, water cleansed in a reciprocal, your Serpentine, and either a small piece of the person's hair, or personal item. If you do not have either, then a virgin white paper to write the person's first and last name upon. You must further ensure that you have your wand upon your person as a means of protection for you as the Practitioner. Set the candle within the offering bowl or dish, next to the personal item or virgin paper, and then light the candle.

Perform widdershins with Serpentine in the left hand, grasped with knuckles upward, hand travelling widdershins around the SAMNU EMUA - Eighth Force – Once the script has been performed, take the hand off the board, to the left, in a sharp motion:

Gi Be Dag Ma Dara Be Ar E Ina Utu, Nanna, Ma Adar Su'ati Annu Piriq Ina Azag Annu Bi Be Sinser Er E Gallas Mamman Aga Azag Bur Annu Aka Annu Wur Eri

Night to be Day and Dark to be Light Raise the sun, moon and star That this the bearer of the magic From the shining bright This command to be twelve to go raise demons Whoever crowns the shining bright hear this divine command This wisdom bind

Now dip the Serpentine into the cleansed water and place onto the Samnu Emua. With your wand in your hand, say these words that follow, and as you say these words, raise your wand from the below to the above:

Gi Be Dag Ma Dara Be Ar A Bana Annu Zipang Antam Ina Ina Arata-Gar Nisme Annu Arazu Agga Alka E Annu Ara Ina Wur Eri

Night to be Day and Dark to be Light I exorcise this spiritual universe From the Earth of the four quarters hear this prayer spirits of the deep Come rise this time in wisdom bind

(Instructions for wand making can be found in the Knights Bible)

Now lower your wand and place on the floor in front of you and kneel down at the dark flame. Raise the personal item (or virgin paper) and burn this as a gift to the Dark Flame One, as you say these words:

Dan Dag Ma Dan Gi Alka Arata-Gar Dura Ama Ma Adda Lu Baru Ma Ara Uru Igara
Mighty Day and Might Night Come the Earth of the four quarters Draw together Mother and Father Let Priest and time guard heron

Now hold your left hand straight, knuckles facing to the above and seal the Samnu Emua (Eighth Force), travelling Deosil as you say these words:

Ei Annu Dar Dir Ma Eri Annu Ina Ara Ma Egir
Exit this Earth land and bind this in time and
future

This is the lesson of the universe, be certain that your performance is just, as to seal the time and bind your thought in prayer; a practice not taken by many.

"However, few may use this Gift of L.i.g.h.t, but
you as one must learn this rite;
To savour all in time to flee, when time and
L.i.g.h.t are here to see."

'Those whom dare to judge shall be judged'

ARAGONITE:

As previously instructed, the Samnu Emua, or Eighth Force is used for one purpose of aligning the healing and magical abilities of the Practitioner to the Recipient. However, we further discovered that it is used for protection and for ritual work. The first learning tool of inner and outer travel; that being the river of stones, is the Aragonite.

It is yours and as long as you have strength to perform and courage to practice, it will guide all practitioners towards the L.i.g.h.t.

This stone has the name Aragonite due to the locality of its truest form, that being Aragon in Spain. However, it should be remembered that this stone has the connection to the Church of St. Mary; the stone will be the K.e.y to your discovery.

Aragonite may be used for healing, but is best placed within the sphere of life, as you will use your thoughts through a life of challenges and discovery. Aragonite is used for travels to the plain of perfection; that place where most dare not travel as those who seek are not always ready to know. It will open your inner thoughts and encourage you to listen to the thoughts of others from within. Let us now perform the script of Namtar, so to charge this stone to you as the holder, making you one with the stone:

THE SCRIPT OF NAMTAR:
(To charge the stone so the practitioner becomes the holder: Performed widdershins with Aragonite in the left hand, grasped with knuckles upward, hand travelling widdershins around the SAMNU EMUA - Eighth Force – Once the script has been performed, take the hand off the board, to the left, in a sharp motion)

Gi Be Dag Ma Dara Be Ar E Ina Utu, Nanna, Ma
Adar Su'ati Annu Piriq Ina Azag Annu Bi Be Sinser
Er E Gallas Mamman Aga Azag Bur Annu Aka
Annu Wur Eri

Night to be Day and Dark to be Light Raise the
sun, moon and star That this the bearer of the
magic From the shining bright This command to
be twelve to go raise demons Whoever crowns
the shining bright hear this divine command This
wisdom bind

You have now charged the Aragonite to you; be
certain in your mind of this caution;

"That the Aragonite charged with Craft in thought
        Must never leave a room once sought,
        A room of time where motions stand
        And stillness within from the inner hand."

OBSODIAN AND HOWLITE:

Charging the Obsidian and Howlite to be as one by the script of Ea (The Messenger – Rakbu)

THE SCRIPT OF EA:

(To charge the stones so the Craft becomes the holder: Performed widdershins with the Obsidian and Howlite in the left hand, grasped with knuckles upward, travelling widdershins around the SAMNU EMUA - Eighth Force – Once the script has been performed, take the hand off the board, to the left, in a sharp motion)

Gi Be Dag Ma Dara Be Ar E Ina Utu, Nanna, Ma Adar Su'ati Annu Piriq Ina Azag Annu Bi Be Sinser Er E Gallas Mamman Aga Azag Bur Annu Aka Annu Wur Eri

Night to be Day and Dark to be Light Raise the sun, moon and star That this the bearer of the magic From the shining bright This command to be twelve to go raise demons Whoever crowns the shining bright hear this divine command This wisdom bind

You have now charged the Obsidian and Howlite as one, a powerful combination.

'When all else fails – Look within to find the solution'

WORKING WITH HERBS & HEALING WITH THE RAKBU DAG:
The secret lore of Alka Antam

You will now discover that the Knight Templar path travels through the realms of combining powers of herbs with sacred stones and for Rites of Passage; the use of candles.

In Templarism these practices are also known as **the Secret Lore of Alka Antam:** i.e. combining the powers of Stones and Herbs by the **Rakbu Dag** (Messenger Chamber)

:

This discovery should not be of light notes; it is the foundation of combining the natural with the supernatural. You will now be introduced to five natural resources within the path; that being:

Hawthorn for Anshar of the north (Moon)
Apple leaf for Lahmu of the east (Venus)
Mandrake root for Anunna of the south (Mars),
Lavender for Kishar of the West (Jupiter)

And the neutral spirit holds:

Lilly leaf for Nabu of the universe (Mercury)

You now need to travel further by ensuring that you understand the true properties and purpose of these natural resources. It is by this knowledge installed (see working chart below) that you are enabled to learn what can be combined, thus to ensure that the spells cast have great impact and outcome. *(important – do not combine more than 3 herbs in any one combination)*

THE MESSENGER CHAMBER: RAKBU DAG

The Messenger Chamber Board can be made of wood, (round breadboards and cork placemats are a very good size) or simply drawn on paper o card, sewn or drawn on to cloth, pyrographed on wood or inscribed upon the ground as shown below:

Also known as the **Rakbu Dag** (Messenger Chamber)

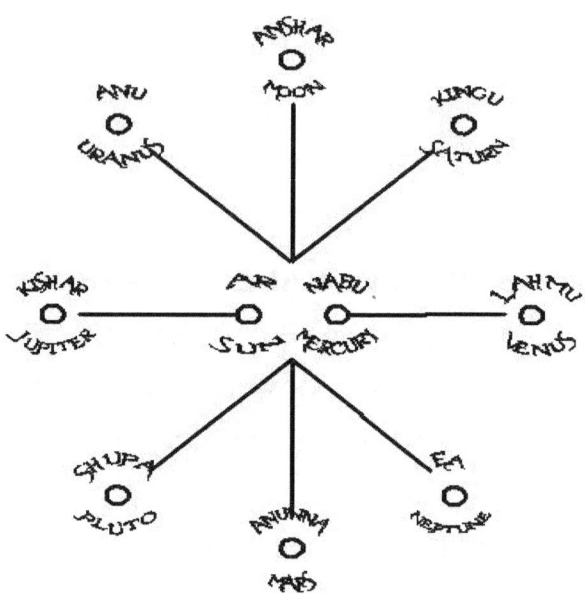

ADVANCEMENT OF HEALING USING THE RAKBU DAG:

You will need the Rakbu Dag (Messenger Chamber) or the Samna Emua (Channel Board), the Sacred Stones, water in a reciprocal, either an individual tea light candle or four tea lights for the compass points, your guide to all sacred stones and the herbs and potions of choice. (see chart above for guidance)

Light a single tea light candle to the left of the Samna Emua, or light four tea light candles at the compass points and choose the herbs/potions to add to your tea light(s). You will need to allow a few minutes for the tea lights to be partly fluid, so to add the herbs and potions of choice.

Cleanse the Water by holding the left hand straight out and with a widdershins (anticlockwise) motion

Urru annu da A dimmu antam, Keezh annu Arazu be Gi ma Dag, wur damu ma bar. Bana gankankha ina ara ma ina ina zagdaku

Guard this gift I order the universe, under this prayer to be night and day, wisdom child and seat of wisdom. Exorcise this vessel in time and in the dark threshold

Have all stones aligned on the Samna Emua or Rakbu Dag within their designated stations and place all other stones upon the board at your choosing. Now hold your Lapis Lazuli tight in your left palm. Raise your hand (Knuckles upwards) over the Channel Board and focus on the energy contained within.

Gently start a Widdershins motion (anti-clockwise) around the board. The speed of the motion is for you to decide, but ensure that all energy attunes to you appropriately. You will know when the stones are ready. Now continue with the Widdershins motion and say this Mystic Chant:

E-gish-shir-gal, E-gish-shir-gal Lu Annu bi ma lalartu eri
House of Great Light, House of Great Light Let this divide and phantom bind

The recipient must now choose two stones, or you may choose the two stones for use in the treatment.

One Stone is chosen for its MAGICAL ABILITY
One stone for its HEALING ABILITY.

Now place both chosen stones into the chalice of water and with your LEFT hand flat, you may perform the Script of Ea, widdershins around the chalice':

Nabu Kur Dingar, E ina Utu, Nanna, ma Adar Su'ati annu Piriq, ina Azag Annu tisa bi er E Gallas Mamman aga Azag bur annu aka annu wur eri

Nabu underworld God, raise the Sun, Moon, and star That this the bearer of the magic, from the shining bright. This ninth command to go raise demons. Whoever crowns the shining bright
Hear this divine command, this wisdom bind

The Recipient now takes the two Sacred Chosen Stones from the chalice and grasps them in their hands as detailed:

The **MAGICAL** ABILITY to be placed in the Recipients **LEFT** Hand.
The **HEALING** ABILITY to be placed in the Recipients **RIGHT** Hand.

The Recipient now lies down on their back, holding the Chosen Stones in the appropriate hands, then releases the stones to naturally fall either in front of the finger tips, or below each palm, whilst lying down.

Now go to the chalice and cleanse you hands as you have been taught in the earlier Degrees and when you feel thoroughly cleansed and charged, start at the top of the Recipient's head and slowly work around the body.

Your hands must not touch the recipient, but flow over the body as long as you feel it is required. You are the only judge in this domain – it is best that your hands flow over the recipients body at about 4 – 10 centimetres away.

Now ask the Recipient to hand you the Sacred Stones, dip them quickly into the chalice of water and place directly back onto the Channel Board. Once again with the LEFT hand and straightened out, move your hand Deosil (Clockwise) around the Channel Board, then quickly off the Board to Seal the Energies.

You have now completed the Psychic Healing with Stones. You must give the tea light (or if you used four tea lights, all four tea lights) to the recipient as a gift for either their continued use, or their disposal.

Be sure to practice well the above healing before moving on, and become familiar with the stones and herbs for your progress to be well founded, commit your heart to your studies and your body to designs.

ADVANCEMENT OF HERB KNOWLEDGE:

It is with great pleasure that the next phase of learning; the advancement of herb knowledge, has been reached; be certain to commit your heart to your studies and your body to designs. For centuries, our ancestors have combined the powers of nature so to nurture the magical properties of this world. You will note that each Deity has more than one herb, and as you will discover in turn, more than one sacred stone to challenge the levels of the magnetic. For now let us cast your focus to the introduction of the advanced properties for your studies.

Needed: A small 'firing sword' (Small heatproof Knight Templar letter opener is fine) which must now be sealed to you. We must do this by lighting the flame of truth (a candle/night-light) and allow a fluid to be born. Once in fluid state add (sparingly) to the liquid:

Black Salt   for the Black Sun of
knowledge

White Salt   for the purification of
wisdom

Mullein Leaf   to attune the
magnetic force of creation

Marjoram   for the purification of
the soul's desire

Now place the Naparu on the floor with sword and
then sprinkle the same combined herbs upon the
floor with the flame of truth (a candle lit). Raise
your hand above the Naparu with your knuckles
upwards as you raise the sword to be as one with
you as you work widdershins (anticlockwise)
around the Naparu:

*A gub annu giral ina ina bulog tia ara. Sahurdub
ina dima zig Ar ma Su.en ma Adar er eri. Redu
ina zi ma kha annu da Ur ma Enlil ma uri ma
esentu. Ba ina annu ara er zig Kima A kha annu
salmu pil billuda*

I cleanse this sword within the circle of time. To raise a cloud of dust in judgement stand. Sun and Moon and Star to bind, to lead the soul and carry this gift. Ground and air and blood and bone, live within this time to stand, as I complete this black flame rite

Now extinguish the flame of truth with the firing sword

You have now completed the charging of the sword to you and with the blessing of the sword and the soul within the fires, you must now prove your understanding of the herbs by producing a herb sachet and a paste of your choosing; be sure to study well and be able to prove on completion why you choose the combinations and whom the gifts are for. As your aid, the full reference library can be found at the front of this book and further charts within this section.

Create your herbal sachets and pastes using the above charts for guidance and once made charge with the following working of the dead:

(Needed are small sachets or pouches, full access to all the herbs listed, olive oil and a pestle and mortar)

Using the charts above and the full listing of herbs, create a herbal sachet for a specific magical or healing purpose, **using no more than three herbs**. Think of what you wish to achieve, your outcome and purpose so to combine the appropriate combination of herbs. The herbal combinations can also be added to olive oil and placed in small pots.

WORKING OF THE DEAD:
This script is to be used to charge the herb sachet or potion you have mixed, prior to its use or presentation to another.

With the sacred stone of Tourmaline (cleansed in the charged water) within your grasp, and with knuckles raised to the above, say the working whilst travelling widdershins (Anticlockwise) around the herb sachet or potion mixed:

Kima A gub annu da Keezh ina Arazu tia Ara Negelta ina walvbane silig Ina bilga ar ma Adar tia dima zig Alka Aradu es Arata ma Lu ba es ushum uri ina zid Ur ma Enlil ma uri ma esentu Qannu tia wur abba ama Bi annu da tia E'Kur ana

As I cleanse this gift under the prayer of time Awake from able shepherd's hand From ancestor light and star of judgement stand Come descend on Earth and let live on dragon blood in truth Ground and air and blood and bone Horn of wisdom elder strong Command this gift of high mound one

You have now charged your Gifts of time for those who are in need and as before practice to become familiar with working with all herbs. At this stage, the knowledge you now have in your grasps will enable you to create a wealth of potions, pouches, candles, ointments and lotions. When practicing healings or just for yourself you may make up an appropriate potion or candle that compliments the healing, for your client to take home. Further more you have the knowledge to make up herb bags and pouches to be worn as a pendant, hung in the home of garden or given as gifts with specific purposes or outcome in mind.

Note: Always prepare and charge as instructed above and use no more than three herbs together; the mixtures can be enhanced by adding the complimentary sacred stone.

NAPARU AND CANDLE MAGIC:

The use of colours within candle magic at this level plays a very significant role, both in the practitioners understanding and evolvement and of a magical use and understanding. We know that colour also refers to specific deities; the understanding of which can be utilised in our practices.

Virgin (new) candles are the most appropriate to use yet during any Black Art Rite we must use black candles. Altar Candles can be re-used as they are cleansed during the opening at each ritual.

The Naparu board is smaller than the Samna Emua and Rakbu Dag yet crafted in the same way and inscribes as shown below:

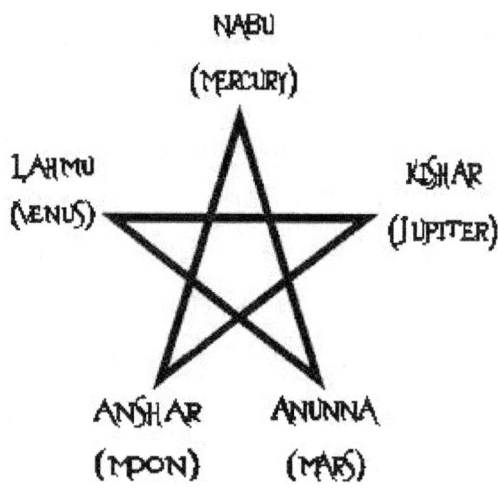

NABU
(MERCURY)

LAHMU
(VENUS)

KISHAR
(JUPITER)

ANSHAR
(MOON)

ANUNNA
(MARS)

North: Howlite (Camphor, Anshar, 30, Moon)
South: Carnelian (Wormwood, Anunna, 3, Mars)
West: Azurite (Honeysuckle, Kishar, 60, Jupiter)
East: Obsidian (Eucalyptus, Lahmu, 50, Venus)
Centre: Jasper (Marshmallow Leaf, Nabu, 60, Mercury)

To continue you will need a small reciprocal for water charged, a small sharp instrument or firing sword for inscribing, your naparu board, a candle of your choice and two herbs/potions of your choice and their associated sacred stones.

Sprinkle (sparingly) the two herbs/potions chosen into the reciprocal then add the water followed by the two chosen associated sacred stones.

You must now cleanse the potion:

Urru annu da A dimmu antam, Keezh annu Arazu be gi ma dag, wur damu ma bar. Bana Gankankha ina ara ma ina ina zagdaku

Guard this gift I order the universe, under this prayer to be night and day, wisdom child and seat of wisdom. Exorcise this vessel in time and in the dark threshold

Once cleansed, pour some of the water into the palm of your hand (does not matter which palm you use) and start to rub your hands up and down the candle. It is important to charge the candle with your own energies, with the thought of the recipient in mind at all times. When cleansing the candle (rub your hands up and down the candle) you must say at low breath:

'Gi be Dag ma Dara be Ar'. Translation: Night to be day and dark to be light

You must now stand the candle upright and light it. Whilst the candle burns, with your forefinger (does not matter whether it be left or right forefinger) wind Deosil (clockwise) around the flame and say:

Ur ma Enlil ma uri ma esentu Qannu tia wur abba ama Bi annu da tia E'Kur ana
Ground and air and blood and bone Horn of wisdom elder strong Command this gift of high mound one

YOU HAVE NOW CHARGED AND PURIFIED YOUR CANDLE.

IT IS NOW TIME TO INSCRIBE OR CARVE INTO THE CANDLE **'NEGELTA'** (AWAKE) FOR SPELL CRAFT

OR **'ZAGDUKU'** (DARK THRESHOLD) FOR HEX CRAFT.

EXTINGUISH THE CANDLE FIRST AND THEN STARTING AT THE TOP AND WORKING DOWN TO THE BOTTOM OF THE CANDLE, YOUR WILL NEED TO CARVE THE CHOSEN DEITY FROM TOP TO BOTTOM, ON THE OPPOSITE SIDE OF YOUR 'NEGELTA' CARVING. THE DEITIES AND PURPOSE ARE LISTED BELOW:

NOTE THAT THERE ARE 8 PRIME COLOURS:
BLACK
RED
WHITE
ORANGE
YELLOW
BROWN
SILVER
BLUE

THE NUMEROLOGY IS SET AS:

50 + 3 + 12 + 30 + 13 + 15 + 40 + 60 + 60 + 60 + 20 + 9 + 5 **= 377**

NOW LET US CONTINUE: 3 + 7 + 7 **= 17**   / **1 + 7 = 8** (THE INFINITY SEQUENCE)

NOW LIGHT YOUR CANDLE ONCE MORE; TRAVEL DEOSIL (CLOCKWISE) AROUND THE FLAME AND SAY:

Bilga pil dim.ti annu es dan ushum igi Uri tia dara ma su tia Arata Dirig bi walv ama
Ina Ara ma edin es samnu er zig Qannu ma esentu alka ina er silig

***Add indicated two lines for **Hex Craft:**

Ina dara er bad er ega eri Annu ezeru tia lu ina silig tia ara Subar annu ezeru ma aradu ina Arata-gar

Ancestor flame retain this on mighty dragon eye Blood of dark and skin of Earth Bow down command be able strong Through time and plain on eighth to stand Horn and bone come through to hand

***From dark to death to dark water bind this curse of man within hand of time Release this curse and descend in the Earth of the four quarters

NOW blow the candle out.

Once extinguished, with the same forefinger you used to raise the energy, you must now wind wider shins (Anti-clockwise) around the candle to contain the powers within (3 times round).

Your gift is now ready. Be sure to instruct the recipient that this is a gift that they must accept. Only they can touch it, and that it must be completely burnt down within 8 weeks or misfortune will fall upon them. If you have raised the candle for Hex Craft then it is you that must burn the candle down yourself.

GENERAL NOTES:

Yellow	Intelligence, Memory, Creativity
Green	Luck and Fertility
Brown	Balance and Focus
Blue	Protection and Wisdom
Pink	Love and Romance
Black	Knowledge and Raising Power
White	Peace and Harmony
Red	Sex, Energy, Health, and courage
Silver	Communication with the Gidim
Orange	To achieve a goal

REFERENCE CHART FOR DEITY/STONE ASSOCIATION IN CANDLE MAGIC

There are Eight Main Birth Colours used for candle magic:

Silver

Black

White

Red

Brown

Orange

Blue

Yellow.

Note that the colour yellow now replaces the colour purple, and as a reference guide below the colour of the candle for Spell cast and a refresher of the Naparu for associated stones:

Positive Energy:

Yellow	Intelligence, Memory, Creativity
Green	Luck and Fertility

Brown	Balance and Focus
Blue	Protection and Wisdom
Pink	Love and Romance
Black	Knowledge and Raising Power
White	Peace and Harmony
Red	Sex, Energy, Health, and courage
Silver	Communication with the Gidim
Orange	To achieve a goal
Purple	Power of the Deities, Material Wealth, High ability to perform magic

Negative Energy:

Yellow	Stupidity, memory, and low mood
Green	Bad luck and infertility
Brown	Imbalance and lack of focus
Blue	To cause ill health

Pink	To destroy love and romance
Black	To drain and steal power(s)
White	To cause war and conflict
Red	To cause bleeding (err side of caution)
Silver	To cause gidim to enter a place
Orange	To cause a fire (err side of caution)
Purple	loss of wealth or halt magical powers

NAPARU STONES WITH CANDLE MAGIC:

Jasper – Nabu – Mercury	Logic and intelligence
Azurite – Kishar – Jupiter	Sexual desire and sexual energy
Carnelian – Anunna – Mars	Courage, power, plague, and war

Howlite – Anshar – Moon   Soul, luck, and
development
Obsidian – Lahmu – Venus   Energy,
travel, stability, and desire

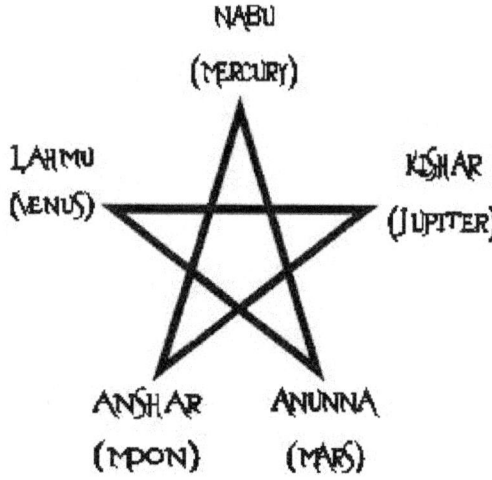

TOURMALINE AND MAGNESITE

We now need to explore the use the Tourmaline
during the ritual of purification upon the entrance
of the nine.

For this purpose you will require the Tourmaline, incense, a small candle, a reciprocal for water charged, sage for purification, lavender to enhance inspiration, raspberry leaf to protect during travel and the Rakbu Dag.

It is important, on this occasion to undertake the purification rite, so to be able to continue to use this working tool (Rakbu Dag) in future practices.

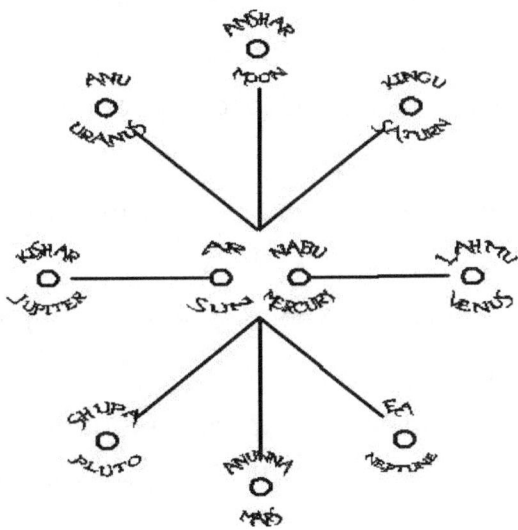

TOURMALINE AND THE NINE:

(Purification Rite: Raising energy from within the nine signs)

For the purpose you will need a candle, your own tourmaline stone, matches, ten pieces of virgin paper, a paper envelope, black salt and white salt, chalice or receptacle with Holy water and your tourmaline, your wand, a chalk spirit stone (or magnesite) and the following potions:

White Willow Bark – Inanna - Purification

White Salt – Nammu - Contractive force in nature

Sage – Nammu - Holy Ghost – Three phases of existence

Marshmallow Leaf – Nabu - Integrative force in nature

Marshmallow Leaf – Nabu – Son – Three phases of existence

Agrimony – Ra.Uban – Expansive force in nature

Olive Oil – Ra.Uban – Father – Three Phases of existence

Travel first around the perimeter sprinkling white salt to the ground widdershins (anticlockwise) saying these words:

Alka gallas tia zagduku ma sibum annu andul Sub Menzug karabu itka ina zag gug ma idu malu Bur annu bi ma apalu annu arazu ina ina samsu Tia ina nigul ar, Ra.Uban, Nabu, ma Nammu

Come demons of dark threshold and witness this protection Cast your blessing upon the boundary seal and know us. Hear this command and answer this prayer in the name Of the everlasting light, Ra.Uban, Nabu, and Nammu

Now cleanses the Holy water– Holding the left hand straight out and with a widdershins – anticlockwise – motion

Urru annu da A dimmu antam, Keezh annu Arazu be Gi ma Dag, wur damu ma bar. Bana gankankha ina ara ma ina ina zagdaku

Guard this gift I order the universe, under this prayer to be night and day, wisdom child and seat of wisdom. Exorcise this vessel in time and in the dark threshold

Now cleanse your hands from the tourmaline chalice filled with Holy water and collect the following: Your wand and a cauldron prepared with black salt within and placed in the centre.

Now draw the following three symbols upon your paper envelope:

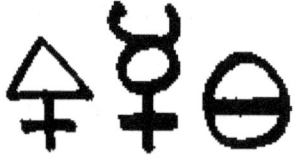

Now place White Willow Bark in the paper envelope to acknowledge Inanna

Now draw each of the following signs onto three separate pieces of virgin paper, and place into the paper envelope:

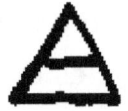

Air: hot and wet

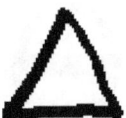

Fire: hot and dry

Water: cold and wet

Note that we are omitting the Earth Sign as this is where we are:

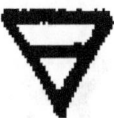

Earth: For cold and dry

Now draw on three separate pieces of virgin paper the 'Three Principles' and add the three principles to the envelope along with their corresponding potion:

(Nammu) Salt: For the contractive force in nature
ADD WHITE SALT

(Ra.Uban) Sulphur: For the expansive force in nature
ADD AGRIMONY

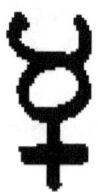

(Nabu) Mercury: Integrative Force of salt and Sulphur

ADD MARSHMALLOW LEAF

Now draw on three separate pieces of virgin paper the 'Three Phases of Existence' and add the three phases to the envelope along with their corresponding potion:

FATHER (Ra.Uban) Olive Oil of the Unknown Master

ADD OLIVE OIL

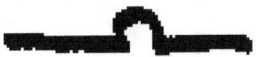

SON (Nabu) Marshmallow Leaf of the Son

ADD MARSHAMALLOW LEAF

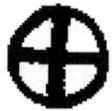

HOLY GHOST (Nammu) Sage of the Holy Ghost
ADD SAGE

TO BECOME AS ONE:

Become seated on the floor your wand in front of you on the floor, when seated comfortably, proceed to ground in a moment of prayer and as you do, close your eyes and bring your hands together in the horned symbol. Focus, with your eyes still closed, on your hands sealed, whilst taking deep slow breathes in and out. Continue with this for a couple of minutes, and when ready open our eyes.

Now place both of your hands into a cup shape, separate them apart (still in a cup shape) by 12.5 centimetres (about 5 inches). Hold the cup shape position and start to rotate your hands in opposite directions by 45 degrees, slowly. Focus on the sixth light of the magnetic force and with your mind's eye focus on the magnetic ball of energy created between your cupped hands.

Continue with this motion and focus on your thoughts of here and now. Focus on the magic you wish to perform on another. When it feels right, from within you, open your cupped hands towards the sky, and as you do, release the magnetic ball and push or blow it towards the sky. Still focusing on the magnetic ball above you in the circle, close your eyes once more and focus on the magic you wish to perform.

THE SCRIPT OF EA: Repeat whilst sitting down and focussing on what you wish your outcome to be.

Nabu kur dingar, E ina Utu, Nanna, ma Adar

Suati annu Piriq, ina azag, annu bi er E gallas

Mamman aga azag bur annu aka, annu wur eri

Nabu underworld God, raise the sun, moon and star That this the bearer of the magic, from the shining bright, this command to go raise demons Whoever crowns the shining bright hear this divine command, this wisdom bind

Now all stand up and commence widdershins (anti-clockwise) motion around your space while repeating the mystic chant:

> *E-gish-shir-gal, E-gish-shir-gal, lu annu bi, ma lalartu eri*

(House of the Great Light, House of the Great Light, let this divide and phantom bind)

Stop the motion and raise your hands toward the above, pause of thought, and bringing your hands down once more. .

Now pick up your wand, still within your space and hold firmly up to the above and say:

Ina wur eri
Through wisdom bind

Now lower your wand when you feel comfortable to do so, be seated for the explanation of the process you have just enacted.

You were sure to cleanse your hands by the **Crystal Chalice**, as no practitioner should perform magic without realigning the energies from within them by ritual cleansing.

A small cauldron was prepared in the centre with black salt so to integrate nature as one. You then created your potion by the signs, or rather by three out of four of the d.o.v.e phases; being:

The Magi

The Three Principles

The Three Phases of Existence

You used a paper envelope to make your potion so to work towards **Becoming as One** and continued to apply the Three Principles by adding:

White Salt for the Holy Ghost, Nammu **to contract nature**

Agrimony for the Father, Ra.Uban **to expand nature**

 Marshmallow Leaf for the Son, Nabu **to integrate nature**

You further expressed your wish with Deity to **Co-exist** by applying the phases, or rather three of the four d.o.v.e phases, by adding:

Olive Oil for the Father, Ra.Uban **to be as one with the serpent for protection**

Marshmallow Leaf for the Son, Nabu **to raise the energies and let through the boundary**

Sage for the Holy Ghost, Nammu **to purify all intentions (good or bad) in balance**

You were seated within the inner circle with your wand to the front, as no witch should ever be seated without the tool of Craft, in readiness from those whom might attack the circle. You were asked to clear your mind and focus by the horned sign as it this stage you were to invoke the aid of Deity to assist you as you enact the ways of times past.

You were asked to cup your hands then separate them about five inches apart, though not realising that you were in fact creating a magnetic sphere, or ball, so to release your thought into the above for power and control of affairs.

You were then asked to release your magnetic sphere toward the above by either pushing or blowing the sphere above you within the inner circle; you then continued to focus before lowering your hands again, for being one of strength you were able to thus absorb the positive and negative forces around you, enabling you to travel freely.

.

You then performed the Script of Ea and although not always necessary, on this occasion it was enacted to seal the energies from all within. You then stood up and raised the power of within to the above by the mystic chant of Great Light and with your mind's eye permitted the spheres you had created to be released onward for their journey. When satisfied that the spheres had commenced their journey, you were encouraged to gather your wands. This final lesson is that by raising your wands upon each other towards the above; your wands enabled channelling of the remaining energy directly into you.

You must now burn your paper pouch by lighting from your candle and placing it into the cauldron

ADVANCEMENT ON THE RAKBU DAG:

For healing in the higher realms/ the secret teachings of the universe to come; working with tourmaline and the messenger chamber

The Rakbu Dag is used in the same way as you Samnu Emua (Eighth Force). However, it is essential to remember that every working tool needs to be charged and raised to become one with you and you one with the tool. In the earlier section you were able to demonstrate your understanding of working with the Samnu Emua and Lapis. On this occasion you will need to demonstrate that you are able to work with the Rakbu Dag and Tourmaline.

Please now align your Rakbu Dag and Sacred Stones together, so to be ready to start:

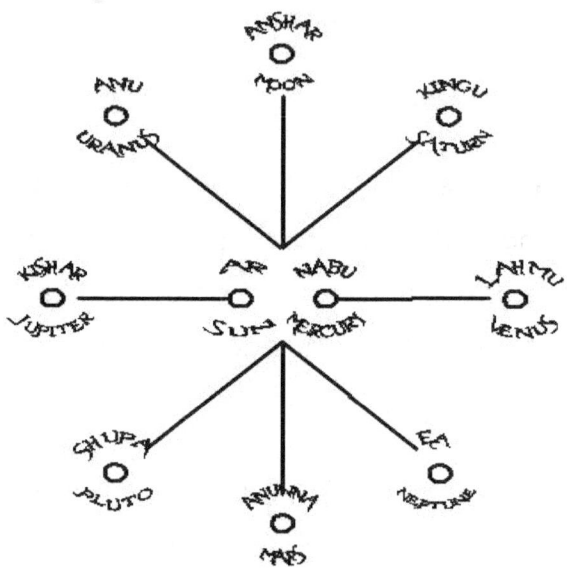

REFERENCE CHART FOR WORKING WITH THE RAKBU DAG

Have all stones aligned on the Channel Board (Rakbu Dag) within their designated stations and place all additional stones (If desired) upon the board at your choosing. Now hold your tourmaline tight in your left palm.

Raise your hand (Knuckles upwards) over the Channel Board and focus on the energy contained within. Gently start a Widdershins motion (anti-clockwise) around the board. The speed of the motion is for you to decide, but ensure that all energy attunes to you appropriately.

You will know when the stones are ready. Now continue with the Widdershins motion and say this Mystic Chant:

E-gish-shir-gal, E-gish-shir-gal Lu Annu bi ma lalartu eri
(House of Great Light, House of Great Light, Let this divide and phantom bind)

*The recipient must now choose two stones, or you may choose the two stones for use in the treatment.

*One Stone is chosen for its **MAGICAL ABILITY**
*The other stone for its **HEALING ABILITY**

Now place both Chosen stones into the chalice of water and with your LEFT hand flat, you may perform the Script of Ea, widdershins around the chalice':

Nabu Kur Dingar, E ina Utu, Nanna, ma Adar Su'ati annu Piriq, ina Azag Annu tisa bi er E Gallas Mamman aga Azag bur annu aka annu wur eri

Nabu underworld God, raise the Sun, Moon, and star That this the bearer of the magic, from the shining bright. This ninth command to go raise demons. Whoever crowns the shining bright. Hear this divine command, this wisdom bind

The Recipient now takes the two Sacred Chosen Stones from the chalice and grasps them in their hands as detailed:

The **MAGICAL ABILITY** to be placed in the Recipient's **LEFT** Hand.

The **HEALING ABILITY** to be placed in the Recipient's **RIGHT** Hand.

The Recipient now lies down on their back, holding the chosen stones in the appropriate hands, then releases the stones to naturally fall either in front of the finger tips, or below each palm, whilst lying down.

Now go to the chalice and cleanse you hands as you have been taught in the earlier section and when you feel thoroughly cleansed and charged, start at the top of the Recipient's head and slowly work around the body.

YOUR HANDS MUST NOT TOUCH THE RECIPIENT, BUT FLOW OVER THE BODY AS LONG AS YOU FEEL IT IS REQUIRED. YOU ARE THE ONLY JUDGE IN THIS DOMAIN – IT IS BEST THAT YOUR HANDS FLOW OVER THE RECIPIENTS BODY AT ABOUT 4 – 10 CENTIMETRES AWAY.

Now ask the Recipient to hand you the Sacred Stones, dip them quickly into the chalice of water and place directly back onto the Channel Board. Once again with the LEFT hand and straightened out, move your hand Deosil (Clockwise) around the Channel Board, then quickly off the Board to Seal the Energies.

You have now completed the healing with session; ensure that the recipient drinks some fluid, as often the recipient will have a sense of dehydration.

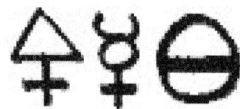

OFFERING FOR USE IN HOLY WATER UPON THE ALTAR: It is now time to make up a paste for your Altar – to use whenever you feel the it is 'right' to add an 'offering' within the Holy Water:

Make up your herbal paste using Marshmallow Leaf, Sage, and Olive Oil. Being the 'Three Principles'

Father – Sulphur – Expand Nature (Substitute: Olive Oil)

Son – Mercury – Integrate Nature (Substitute: Marshmallow Leaf)

Holy Ghost – Salt – Contract Nature (Substitute: Sage)

Keep your paste well, and do not use it liberally.

A connection to the Land:

Within our Path we have direct connections not only to the land, but also to the spirits within, and around us. Such spirits exist within living things, be it trees, oceans, or wildlife. This will be an ongoing exploration as you establish your connections to the land and life as one.

Before the Great Flood that cleansed the world, the Priests of ancient Lemuria; the civilization of which were deeply religious and spiritually connected to the land; In order to preserve their knowledge, the priest were sent out to travel the world in order to spread their knowledge with as many civilizations as they could reach. The priests further stored their wisdom and knowledge within Sacred Stones; or rather crystals that would be hidden in underground tunnels, deep within the Earth. The Priests believed that by spreading the word of the land and storing the wisdom and knowledge within Sacred Stones, that the information would never be forgotten, that it would be retained within the DNA of humans and passed down. The Priests further believed that the Sacred Stones, or the rather the stones and the Me, would be found in future lifetimes, but only at a perfect point in time would the stones and the Me be discovered.

The Priests created detailed maps of the magnetic grid of the Earth, and it was at these perfect points that they preserved the stones, and at the central point, the preservation of the Me. The locations of the magnetic grid of the Earth were passed down to their sons and daughters for seven thousand years, though it is important to distinguish that a person being referred to as a son or daughter is not necessarily a biological offspring, but rather in the sense of a teacher to the student

There are several 'perfect points' around the globe were the energy alignments are extremely powerful; where the energy of the stars and the energy of the earth align., but it is important to focus on energies as a whole and working with sacred stones especially quartz.

We know that quartz holds information and knowledge of Lemuria. Many peoples around the globe today, still have access to this ancient knowledge, but for many thousands of years the peoples of this planet have not been ready for this hidden information.

It is said that the time of the Awakening is drawing near for those who truly 'see'; those in tune with the 'within' and 'without' and to the vibrational energies of sacred stones and to the rejuvenating energies of the Earth itself

'Ah Isle of Rubble where ends a freeman's court.
Inscribed as Adam half my clues consort'

.

SACRED WATER OF TIME: Remember well, for you are now able to create the sacred water of time within the chalice of life by holding within the chalice - Water Cleansed, Salt, Myrrh:

By using this combination during travel for cleansing, your inner light will open with fulfilment.

INFINITY TRANCE: 'THE GENERATION OF LIFE'

The Infinity Trance is a term used for the generation of the energy of life. When you, or others feel low, or perhaps just wish to raise the cone of power, then this particular trance should be enacted to enrich recipients and requires only the seal of time to proceed.

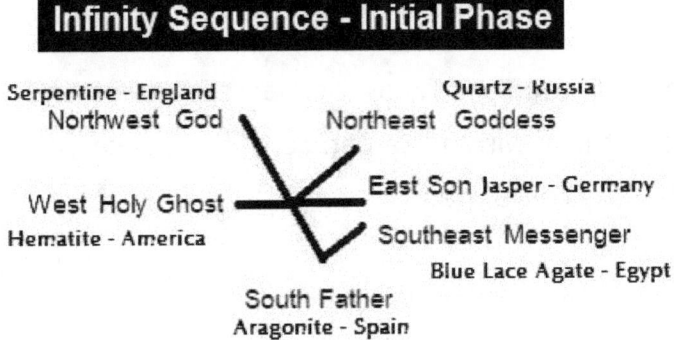

Using the above sequence, you must first create your potions and place at the magnetic points, with a candle, for examples:

Northwest	God
Northeast	Goddess
West	Holy Ghost
East	Son
South	Father
Southeast	Messenger

You will need the following Sacred Stones and place them within the centre of the space you wish to create, namely:

Northwest   God

     Serpentine – England

Northeast   Goddess

     Quartz – Russia

West   Holy Ghost

     Hematite – America

East   Son

     Jasper – Germany

South   Father

     Aragonite – Spain

Southeast   Messenger

     Blue Lace Agate – Egypt

You will further need to place the following potions to the centre:

- 🕐 Burdock Root, Hawthorn, Camphor, White Willow, Raspberry Leaf and Sage

- 🕐 For each participant, a tea light candle will be required:

🕐 Place the tea light candle to the centre

🕐 For each participant, an incense cone or stick will be required:

🕐 Place the incense (Preferably Nag Champa) to the centre

🕐 You will require the Trinity Potion to be placed at the centre:

Father – Olive Oil
Son – Marshmallow Leaf
Holy Ghost – Sage

You will require Salt and Myrrh combined:
Mix Salt and Myrrh with Holy Water.

The centre must now be prepared with the Cauldron Potion: Burdock Root, Hawthorn, Camphor, White Willow, Raspberry Leaf, and Sage.

Once added to the cauldron, take long deep breaths and say these words:

Negelta ina ina rebu emua pil, bilga tia ina salmu ar Aradu es annu dag, ma apalu annu Billuda subar ina zi, nisme annu bi ma de zid da ig.igi, ma idu su'ati mamman zig subar duramah. Zig kha da ana

Awake from the fourth force flame, ancestors of the black sun descend on this chamber and answer this rite to release the soul. Hear this command and carry truth with those who see and know that whoever stands to release the Great Stag stands complete with one

Now pour the water into the Cup of Life and raise the energy within with your hand straight and knuckles upwards:

Left hand straight out and widdershins – anticlockwise – motion

Urru annu da A dimmu antam, Keezh annu Arazu be Gi ma Dag, wur damu ma bar. Bana gankankha ina Ara ma ina ina zagdaku

Guard this gift I order the universe, under this prayer to be night and day, wisdom child and seat of wisdom. Exorcise this vessel in time and in the dark threshold

Now place the Sacred Stones into the Cup of Life, in the following sequence, and say these words:

Alka ina ina gidim quannu duramah, gibil wur, su'ati zae da. Durisam ina karabu ma sibum annu da er ina antam

Come through the spirit horn the great stag, one of fire wisdom, that you make forever this blessing and witness this offering to the universe. May this Cup of Life hold the key to eternal freedom through Ilu, Amalug, Nammu, Nabu, Ra.uban and Rakbu

Ilu	Northwest	God
	Serpentine – England	
Amalug	Northeast	Goddess
	Quartz – Russia	
Nammu	West	Holy Ghost
	Hematite – America	
Nabu	East	Son
	Jasper – Germany	
Ra.uban	South	Father
	Aragonite – Spain	
Rakbu	Southeast	
Messenger	Blue Lace Agate– Egypt	

Now take a small sip of the water as you say these words:

Ina muh tia ti ina ar enmen nu
The Cup of Life through time thirst not

Add the Trinity Potion to the Salt and Myrrh, then proceeds to anoint yourself on the forehead as below while repeating the words:

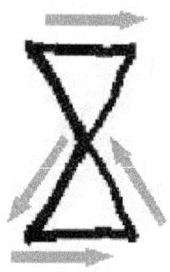

A gug annu itka zae ina ina sa tia ina Adda, ina Ban, ma ina Kuggal Alad
I seal this upon you in the name of the Father, the Son, and the Holy Ghost

Travel to the centre light a candle and then the incense cone or stick, and say:

Anamea (An-a-me-a) ma nigul (Nig-ul)
Everything and everlasting

Once complete, they return back to form a circle once more and re-link hands
Participants now hum at low breath (softly hum) the word of peace until it feels right to stop:

Inimdug (In-im-dug) - Peace

Proceed to walk around the circle Deosil (clockwise) chanting the words below:

Uri ma Esentu - Uri ma Esentu - Ala ina ara Mupad kima esdu

Then travel widdershins (anti-clockwise), slowly to start, then gaining speed as the chant develops.

Blood and Bone - Blood and Bone - All in time to invoke as one

When it feels right to stop the circle motions, do so.

Now travel widdershins sprinkling 'salt and myrrh' repeating these words:

Uri ma Esentu - Uri ma Esentu - Ala ina ara Mupad kima esdu

When finished, stop at this point, close your eyes and focus on your inner thoughts, open eyes and when ready break the circle.

At this point extinguish the central candle and dip the incense into the 'Cup of Life' (If still burning) but be certain to practice the above when solitary until familiar.

'In the month of May I saw a tremendous light that brightened the skies as it ventured toward Earth. Little was known of the impact that was about to occur'

MAGNESITE, SUNSTONE AND OPALITE:

MAGNESITE: 'THE CHALK SPIRIT STONE'

The Chalk Spirit Stone or Magnesite is the next stone, within our path of L.I.G.H.T, to explore the purpose of. The full exploration of Magnesite can be found within the complete listing of herbs and stones. Take note, that from hereon, Sacred Stones will be in collective form and more importantly, of a collective use.

Now that the introduction to this magnificent stone is concluded, you must now charge this stone to be personal to you. This is undertaken with a different strategy to your studies to date. For this exercise you will require a small cauldron, Agrimony, three clear quartz crystals, a candle and Holy water.

Charging Magnesite for personal use:
Working Tools: Cauldron, Agrimony,   Magnesite, Three pieces of clear Quartz, A Candle, Holy Water

Working Script: *Uri ma esentu, uri ma esentu, Ala ina ara mupad kima esdu*

Blood and bone, blood and
bone,

All in time to invoke as one

Instruction:

- ⏱ Place the cauldron in front of you
- ⏱ Sprinkle enough Agrimony, so to cover the bottom of the cauldron
- ⏱ Place the three pieces of clear quartz into the centre of the cauldron
- ⏱ Now cleanse your hands with the Holy water, as you have previously been instructed
- ⏱ Pick up your Magnesite and place it inside the cauldron
- ⏱ Now light your candle (this should be to the side of the cauldron) and say the 'working script'
- ⏱ Focus your eyes on the candle, whilst taking long, deep breaths

- As you continue to focus upon the candle alight, start to tune into the space around you, as you feel a connection to all in space and time
- When it feels right to do so, extinguish the candle and say these words: *Sugid annu kima ina shahar tia ala girius ina ar tia zid Accept this as the beginning of a step upon the light of truth*
- Now retract the Magnesite from the cauldron – It is yours to keep until your time of passing

SUNSTONE AND THE MAGNETIC SEQUENCE:

This sacred stone has the energy alignment of the stars and is a stone of the Goddess path.

Previously you were shown a sequence and were provided with the introduction of Sacred Stones within:

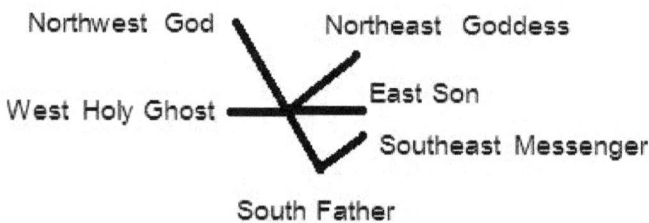

The Magnetic Sequence of Time

Northwest God   Northeast Goddess

West Holy Ghost   East Son

Southeast Messenger

South Father

Note: God, Goddess, and Messenger (Judges)
Father, Son, Holy Ghost (Divine Trinity)

However, there was a missing link within this formation; being the central core of the sequence; that being the Sunstone. Let us first explore the Sunstone, before we venture onto the Rite of Passage of the sequence in time. Please refer to the complete Sacred Stone listings for further info on Sunstone

Charging Sunstone for personal use:

Working Tools: Cauldron, Myrrh, Sunstone, Three pieces of clear Quartz,   A Candle, Holy Water

Working Script: *Uri ma esentu, uri ma esentu,*
    Ala ina ara mupad kima esdu
    Blood and bone, blood and
bone,
    All in time to invoke as one

Instruction:

- Place the cauldron in front of you
- Sprinkle a small amount of myrrh into the bottom of the cauldron
- Place the three pieces of clear quartz into the centre of the cauldron
- Now cleanse your hands with the Holy water, as you have previously been instructed
- Pick up your Sunstone and place it inside the cauldron
- Now light your candle (this should be to the side of the cauldron) and say the 'working script'
- Focus your eyes on the candle, whilst taking long, deep breaths

- As you continue to focus upon the candle alight, start to tune into the space around you, as you feel a connection to all in space and time
- When it feels right to do so, extinguish the candle and say these words: Sugid annu kima ina shahar tia ala girius ina ar tia zid Accept this as the beginning of a step upon the light of truth
- Now retract the Sunstone from the cauldron – It is yours to keep until your time of passing

Now that you have your Magnesite of the God and your Sunstone, an aspect of the Goddess, it is time to align the sequence of time.

You will need the following Sacred Stones:

Northeast   Goddess
        Sunstone – Norway
Northeast   Goddess
        Quartz – Russia
Northwest   God
        Magnesite – Brazil

Northwest   God

       Serpentine – England

West   Holy Ghost

       Hematite – America

East   Son

       Jasper – Germany

South   Father

       Aragonite – Spain

Southeast   Messenger

       Blue Lace Agate – Egypt

You will further need to place the following potions to the centre:
Burdock Root, Hawthorn, Camphor, White Willow, Raspberry Leaf, and Sage

One tea light candle will be required:
Place the tea light candle to the centre

An incense cone or stick will be required:
Place the incense (Preferably Nag Champa) to the centre

You will require the Trinity Potion to be placed at the centre:
Father – Olive Oil
Son – Marshmallow Leaf
Holy Ghost – Sage

You will require Salt and Myrrh combined:
Mix Salt and Myrrh with Holy Water

The centre must now be prepared with the Cauldron Potion:
Burdock Root, Hawthorn, Camphor, White Willow, Raspberry Leaf and Sage – Once added to the cauldron, say these words:

Now say these words:

Negelta ina ina rebu emua pil, bilga tia ina salmu ar Aradu es annu dag, ma apalu annu Billuda subar ina zi, nisme annu bi ma de zid da ig.igi, ma idu su'ati mamman zig subar duramah. Zig kha da ana

Awake from the fourth force flame, ancestors of the black sun descend on this chamber and answer this rite to release the soul. Hear this command and carry truth with those who see and know that whoever stands to release the Great Stag stands complete with one

Pour the water into the 'Cup of Life' – Raise energy within:

Left hand straight out - Knuckles upwards – Widdershins – anticlockwise – motion

Urru annu da A dimmu antam, Keezh annu Arazu be Gi ma Dag, wur damu ma bar. Bana gankankha ina Ara ma ina ina zagdaku

Guard this gift I order the universe, under this prayer to be night and day, wisdom child and seat of wisdom. Exorcise this vessel in time and in the dark threshold

Place the Sacred Stones into the Cup of Life and say these words:

Alka ina ina gidim quannu duramah, gibil wur, su'ati zae da Durisam ina karabu ma sibum annu da er ina antam

Come through the spirit horn the great stag, one of fire wisdom, that you make forever this blessing and witness this offering to the universe. May this Cup of Life provide the key to eternal freedom through Amalug, Ilu and Rakbu

Northeast   Goddess
        Sunstone – Norway
Northeast   Goddess
        Quartz – Russia
Northwest   God
        Magnesite – Brazil
Northwest   God
        Serpentine – England
West   Holy Ghost
        Hematite – America

East	Son
Jasper – Germany	
South	Father
Aragonite – Spain	
Southeast	Messenger
Blue Lace Agate – Egypt	

Now drink from the Cup of Life and say these
words:

Ina muh tia ti ina ar enmen nu
The Cup of Life through time thirst not

Add the Trinity Potion to the salt and myrrh, then
cleanse your hands as you have been instructed.
Anoint upon your forehead as follows:

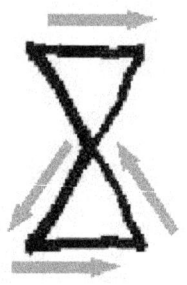

Ina ina sa tia ina Kuggal Alad, Ban, ma
ina Adda
In the name of the Holy Ghost, Son,
and the Father

Light the Incense as say these words:

Anamea (An-a-me-a) ma nigul (Nig-ul) Inimdug
(In-im-dug)
Everything and everlasting peace
Uri ma esentu, uri ma esentu ala in ara mupad
kima esdu
Blood and bone, blood and bone, all in time to
invoke as one

At this stage lay down upon the floor. Close your eyes and focus upon your breathing and circulation. Be certain to focus on these two aspects only, for this is your time and the place to clear your mind of all emotion and all things earthly.

 *Allow yourself time to relax and unwind – continuously focusing on slowing your breathing and slowing your circulation – A maximum of five minutes should be given for the first few attempts, then increase the time to a maximum of fifteen minutes.

When ready – regulate your breathing and circulation. When fully regulated and recharged bring yourself back to this plain and open your eyes.

Take a few moments to feel that you are fully back within this space.

Extinguish your candle, and say these words:

Inimdug ina ara - Peace in time

Before you can move to the next stage within this Art, you will need to ensure that you master the Art of Regulation, the Art of attuning to all things natural, so to break the chains, to work within the supernatural. Take time to develop this skill; for to be classed as worthy amongst us.

WORKING WITH OPALITE (OPAL):

At this stage of your progress towards the L.i.g.h.t, you have embraced the hidden knowledge of the stones and how such knowledge has empowered you to move ever onward. It is therefore the time of passage to explore the use of Opalite, a semi-precious stone, and how such an object empowers the Practitioner to look within so to be without; a subject area that is explored in greater depth within The Knights Bible. Opalite is used as a means of association, that ultimate connection to the life force within you and the universal aspects of the One. It is the fundamental creation of existence, as we must learn to be without – so to be within the spheres of time. It is the composition of the Messenger, in true form of Moss Opalite, being able to remove energy blockages to awaken the third eye of the mind. Being introduced in Hong Kong to the public at large in 1988, its composition has left many in a state of curiosity. It is a semi-precious stone due to its human interference, yet in raw forms the alchemical transformation is considered a key aspect of understanding. Please refer to the complete Sacred Stone listings for further info on Opalite.

Charging Opalite (Opal) for personal use:

Working Tools: Cauldron, Mugwort, Opalite (Opal), Three pieces of clear Quartz, A Candle, Holy Water

Working Script: *Uri ma esentu, uri ma esentu,*
Ala ina ara mupad kima esdu
Blood and bone, blood and
bone,
All in time to invoke as one

- ⏀ Instruction:
- ⏀ Place the cauldron in front of you
- ⏀ Sprinkle a small amount of Mugwort into the bottom of the cauldron
- ⏀ Place the three pieces of clear quartz into the centre of the cauldron
- ⏀ Now cleanse your hands with the Holy water, as you have previously been instructed

- ⏱ Pick up your Opalite (Opal) and place it inside the cauldron
- ⏱ Now light your candle (this should be to the side of the cauldron) and say the 'working script'
- ⏱ Focus your eyes on the candle, whilst taking long, deep breaths
- ⏱ As you continue to focus upon the candle alight, start to tune into the space around you, as you feel a connection to all in space and time
- ⏱ When it feels right to do so, extinguish the candle and say these words: *Sugid annu kima ina shahar tia ala girius ina ar tia zid Accept this as the beginning of a step upon the light of truth*
- ⏱ Now retract the Opalite (Opal) from the cauldron – It is yours to keep until your time of passing

Now that you have your Opalite (Opal), an aspect of the Messenger, it is time to focus upon the stone through the sphere of knowledge, the Crystal Ball.

COMMENCE SPHERE OPENING SEQUENCE OF TIME:

This will be your first step in working with the crystal ball, and although a short time will be spent at this time, it is expected that you will learn to master the art of this working tool in time to come.

Place the Crystal Ball within the centre of the space:

The Crystal ball will represent the sphere of time. Stand in front of the sphere with your Opalite (Opal) in your LEFT hand.

Recipient closes eyes and takes long, deep, slow breaths:

Now close your eyes and take long, deep, slow breaths as you focus in your minds eye upon the sphere of time placed within the centre of knowledge.

Before commencing chant cast white salt around the perimeter of the space

Start the Opening Phase:
Whilst standing firm, commence the opening phase of the raising chant collective, at low breath, the Phase of peace, and continue this until it feels linked in time:

Recipients: *'Inimdug'* Chant (Peace)
Now start to move in a widdershins motion (anti-clockwise) around the space, with your eyes wide open – but within your mind's eye, focus upon the sphere of time (the crystal ball within the centre of your space

Continue travelling widdershins (anti-clockwise) then start the blood and bone chant, and once rotations are in sequence; travel Deosil (clockwise), with the second phase of the opening:

Chant First Stage:
Uri ma Esentu, Uri ma Esentu
Ala ina ara Mupad Kima esdu
Blood and Bone, Blood and Bone
All in time to invoke as one

Chant Second Stage:
Ki ma An, Ki ma An
Eri kima ana, Da gar Sargad
Earth and Sky, Earth and Sky
Bind as one, with four worlds

Now slow your motion until stationery once more and be seated upon the floor facing the sphere of time. Focus on the sphere and let your mind open the sphere to your thoughts

CONTINUE WITH THIRD PHASE OF OPENING:

Se tia Atuku (At-Uk-U)

Cone of Power

Tribal Chant commences and continues for five minutes

Now bring your mind back to the here and now and spend a moment with the connection to your Opalite (Opal).

This is as you need to travel in this stage of your understanding of herbs and crystals, but with this true form of Crystal and Herb Magic reference guide for your practice and use, please take time to study and practice this Art before moving on.

"What secrets do they long to tell
Within your mind where magic dwells?"

QUICK REFERENCE FOR SACRED STONE & HERBAL MAGIC:

HEALING & OPENING OF THE VEIL:

Amalug – 15 – Goddess – Snake (Sibbu) – Holy Ghost – Without - White – Northeast – Mary Magdalene – Sword

Ilu – 30 – God – Ram (Puhalu) – Father – Within - Black – Northwest – Jesus of Nazareth – Stone

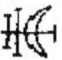

Nabu – 60 – The Me: Us – Hawk (Pag) – Human - Red – Southwest – The Green Man: Jul – Chalice

Mulan – 3 – Future – Goat (Durah) – Star - Grey – South – Future Star – Working Tool of Insight

Rakbu – 12 – Messenger – Wolf (Urbara) – Magical Art - Blue – Southeast – John the Baptist – Spear / Wand

STONE REFERENCE:
Amalug: 15 – Goddess – Snake (Sibbu) – Holy Ghost – Without - White – Northeast – Mary Magdalene – Sword.

Howlite - America

Clear Quartz - Russia

Hematite - America

Moonstone - Sri Lanka

Lapis Lazuli - Afghanistan

Tourmaline - Brazil

Dark Amber - Poland

Malachite - Siberia

Sunstone – Norway

.

Ilu: 30 – God – Ram (Puhalu) – Father – Within - Black – Northwest – Jesus of Nazareth – Stone.

Carnelian – Brazil

Aragonite - Spain

Magnesite - Brazil

Smokey Quartz - Scotland

Nabu: 60 – The Me: Us – Hawk (Pag) – Human - Red – Southwest – The Green Man: Jul – Chalice.

Opalite/Opal – Australia

Azurite - South Africa

Onyx - Brazil

Fire Opal – Mexico

Mulan: 3 – Future – Goat (Durah) – Star - Grey – South – Future Star – Working Tool of Insight.

Tigers Eye - South Africa

Jasper – Germany

Moldavite – Czech Republic

Amethyst – India

Tektite (with sandstone) – China.

Rakbu; 12 – Messenger – Wolf (Urbara) – Magical Art - Blue – Southeast – John the Baptist – Spear/Wand.

Blue Lace Agate – Egypt

Obsidian – Japan Serpentine - England

Citrine – Brazil

Calcite – America.

HERB REFERENCE:

Amalug: 15 – Goddess – Snake (Sibbu) – Holy Ghost – Without - White – Northeast – Mary Magdalene – Sword.

Burdock Root

Hawthorn

Camphor

Raspberry Leaf

Sage

Mullein Leaf

Rosemary

Frankincense

Lavender.

Ilu: 30 – God – Ram (Puhalu) – Father – Within - Black – Northwest – Jesus of Nazareth – Stone.

Wormwood

Kelp

Olive leaf and Oil

Agrimony.

Nabu; 60 – The Me: Us – Hawk (Pag) – Human - Red – Southwest – The Green Man: Jul – Chalice.

Marjoram

Marshmallow Leaf

Apple Leaf

Eucalyptus

Mugwort

Honeysuckle

Myrrh

Mulan: 3 – Future – Goat (Durah) – Star - Grey – South – Future Star – Working Tool of Insight.

White Willow Bark,

Rakbu: 12 – Messenger – Wolf (Urbara) – Magical Art - Blue – Southeast – John the Baptist – Spear / Wand.

Holly Leaf

Lily Leaf

Mandrake Root.

Please refer to the complete Sacred Stone and Herb listings at the front of the book for further info on all of the above Stones and Herbs.

NAPARU ASCENSION:

Sequence for Healing: You will have noticed that as you have made progress and advancement through the levels of healing; that the sequences for the alignment of stones on the healing boards have changed too. Each stage advances the practitioner to a higher level of practice to discover some of the hidden mysteries of magic. It is important to practice at each level and to tune into the 'energies' of the boards; each alignment of stones is different as the energies/magnetics become more powerful as the student progresses and it is important to tune into these energies. Not only are you tuning into the energies of alignments/of the universe but you are attuning yourself too.

We started with the following sequence for the Naparu:

Naparu Cipher

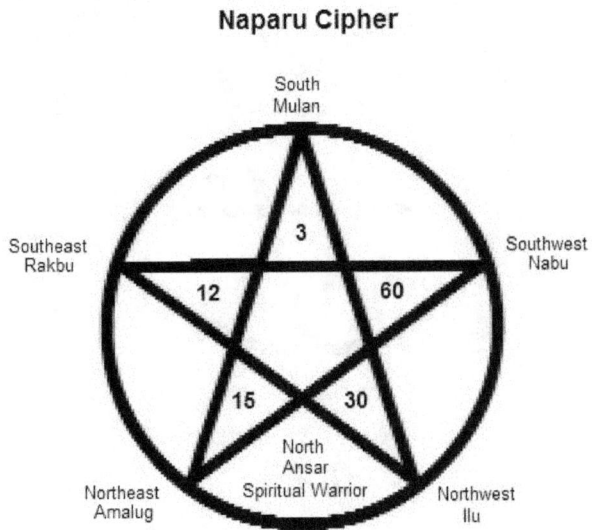

And at this next stage, we will progress to the Naparu Ascension, using the below sequence:

Naparu Ascension

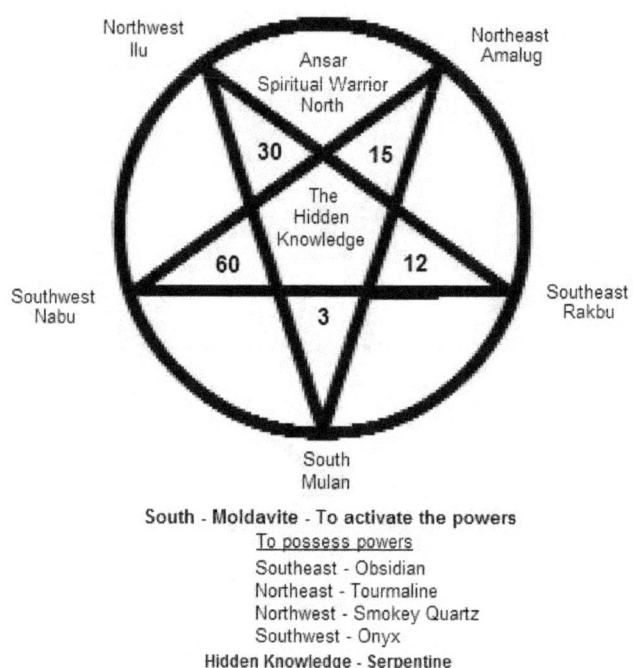

South - Moldavite - To activate the powers
To possess powers
Southeast - Obsidian
Northeast - Tourmaline
Northwest - Smokey Quartz
Southwest - Onyx
Hidden Knowledge - Serpentine

By using the Hidden Knowledge of the Serpent Priesthood (Egyptian Mysteries) we are able (permitted) to walk upon the saddled shores of time.

CHARGING OF SACRED STONES FOR PERSONAL USE:

Working Tools: Cauldron, *Herb of the associated Energy, *Sacred Stone, Three pieces of clear Quartz, A Candle, Holy Water

Working Script: *Uri ma esentu, uri ma esentu, Ala ina ara mupad kima esdu - Blood and bone, blood and bone, All in time to invoke as one*

1. **Instruction:**
2. Place the cauldron in front of you
3. Sprinkle a small amount of <*herb*> into the bottom of the cauldron
4. Place the three pieces of clear quartz into the centre of the cauldron
5. Now cleanse your hands with the Holy water, as you have previously been instructed
6. Pick up your <*sacred stone*> and place it inside the cauldron

7. Now light your candle (this should be to the side of the cauldron) and say the 'working script'

8. Focus your eyes on the candle, whilst taking long, deep breaths

9. As you continue to focus upon the candle alight, start to tune into the space around you, as you feel a connection to all in space and time

10. When it feels right to do so, extinguish the candle and say these words: Sugid annu kima ina shahar tia ala girius ina ar tia zid Accept this as the beginning of a step upon the light of truth

11. Now retract the *<sacred stone>* from the cauldron – It is yours to keep until your time of passing

SACRED STONE HEALING (CRYSTAL HEALING)

You will need your Naparu ascension, (cloth, board, paper, stone or slate), your K.e.y stones, your Sacred Stones, and a chalice filled with water. Have all stones aligned upon the Naparu Ascension within their designated alignment and place all additional stones (If desired) upon the board at your choosing. Now hold your Serpentine tight in your left palm. Raise your hand (Knuckles upwards) over the Naparu Ascension and focus on the energy contained within. Charge the Cup of Life and raise the energy within. With your hand straight and knuckles upward: Left hand straight out and widdershins – anticlockwise – motion

Urru annu da A dimmu antam, Keezh annu Arazu be Gi ma Dag, wur damu ma bar. Bana gankankha ina Ara ma ina ina zagdaku
Guard this gift I order the universe, under this prayer to be night and day, wisdom - child and seat of wisdom. Exorcise this vessel in time and in the dark threshold

Gently start a widdershins motion (anti-clockwise) around the Naparu Ascension. The speed of the motion is for you to decide, but ensure that all energy attunes to you appropriately. You will know when the stones are ready. Now continue with the widdershins motion and say this Mystic Chant:

E-gish-shir-gal, E-gish-shir-gal Lu Annu bi ma lalartu eri
House of Great Light, House of Great Light Let this divide and phantom bind

Recipient must now choose two stones, or you may choose the two stones for use in the treatment.

One Stone is chosen for its **Magical ability (left)** And the other stone for its **Healing ability (right)**

Now place both Chosen stones into the chalice of water and with your LEFT hand flat, you may perform the Script of the Red Spirits, widdershins around the chalice:

Nabu Kur Dingar, E ina Utu, Nanna, ma Adar Su'ati annu Piriq, ina Azag Annu tisa bi er E Gallas Mamman aga Azag bur annu aka annu wur eri

Nabu underworld God, raise the Sun, Moon, and star That this the bearer of the magic, from the shining bright This ninth command to go raise demons Whoever crowns the shining bright Hear this divine command, this wisdom bind

Recipient now takes the two Sacred Chosen Stones from the chalice and grasps them in their hands as detailed:

Left hand for **Magical** ability.
Right hand for **Healing** ability.

The Recipient now lies down on their back, holding the Chosen Stones in the appropriate hands, then releases the stones to naturally fall either in front of the finger tips, or below each palm, whilst lying down. Now go to the chalice and cleanse you hands as you have been taught, and when you feel thoroughly cleansed and charged, start at the top of the Recipient's head and slowly work around the body.

YOUR HANDS MUST NOT TOUCH THE RECPIENT, BUT FLOW OVER THE BODY FOR AS LONG AS YOU FEEL IT IS REQUIRED. YOU ARE THE ONLY JUDGE OF THIS DOMAIN – IT IS BEST THAT YOUR HANDS FLOW OVER THE RECPIENTS BODY AT ABOUT 4 – 10 CENTOIMETRES AWAY.

Once complete, the Recipient must hand you the Sacred Stones, dip them quickly into the chalice of water and place directly back onto the Naparu Ascension. Once again with the *left* hand straightened out, move your hand Deosil (Clockwise) around the Naparu Ascension, then quickly off the Board to seal the Energies. You have now completed the healing with session – Ensure that the recipient drinks some fluid, as often have a sense of dehydration

Charge water
Charge the Cup of Life and raise the energy within
With your hand straight and knuckles upward: Left hand straight out and widdershins – anticlockwise – motion

Urru annu da A dimmu antam, Keezh annu Arazu be Gi ma Dag, wur damu ma bar. Bana gankankha ina Ara ma ina ina zagdaku

Guard this gift I order the universe, under this prayer to be night and day, wisdom - child and seat of wisdom. Exorcise this vessel in time and in the dark threshold

- North – Ansar – Journey of the Spiritual Warrior
- Northeast – Amalug – Goddess and Corner Stone
- Southwest – Nabu – The Me – Time, Sons / Daughters
- Southeast – Rakbu – The Messenger
- Northwest – Ilu – The G.O.D – Universe to Come
- North – Ansar – Return to find within
- South – Mulan – Ascension – The Future Star

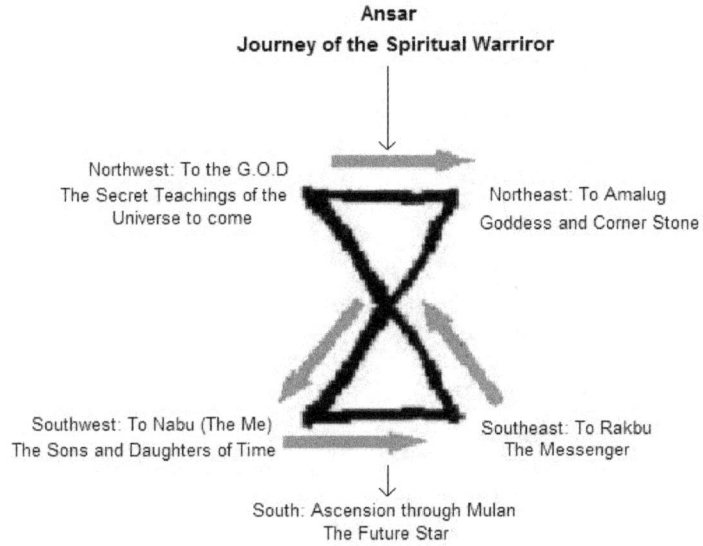

Ansar
Journey of the Spiritual Warriror

Northwest: To the G.O.D
The Secret Teachings of the
Universe to come

Northeast: To Amalug
Goddess and Corner Stone

Southwest: To Nabu (The Me)
The Sons and Daughters of Time

Southeast: To Rakbu
The Messenger

South: Ascension through Mulan
The Future Star

Herbal Trinity – Potion of Protection

Anamea (An-a-me-a) ma nigul (Nig-ul)
Everything and everlasting

> *Uri ma esentu*
> *Blood and Bone*
> *Uri Ma Esentu*
> *Blood and Bone*

Ala ina ara

All in time

Mupad kima esdu

to invoke as one

Ki ma An

Earth and Sky

Ki ma An

Earth and Sky

Eri kima ana

Bind as one

Da gar Sargad

With four worlds

Trinity Potion:

Sulphur – Expand Nature (Substitute: Olive Oil)

Mercury – Integrate Nature (Substitute: Marshmallow Leaf)

Salt – Contract Nature (Substitute: Sage)

VOODOO: A PRACTICAL GUIDE

Voodoo is the modern term used for the practice of a magical art. However, it should be noted that in its raw form the term 'Vodun' (Fon Language meaning God or Spirit) is more specific to the Rites. The origin of Voodoo is IN 'Benin', West Africa – Note that there are elements of Masonic Rituals contained within the ceremonies (rituals). The ancient African worship of the Loa is through possession and chants or dancing around the Poteau-mitan is certain to reveal an experience for all. Worshippers undertake this ritual until the Loa possesses one of them.

STRUCTURE OF VOODOO:

Bondye: Grand Master (Not worshipped on the earthly Plain)

Loa: Demon (Gallas) – Note that Demons practice is good or bad

The Dead: Collective Ancestral Spirits

Asogwe: Supreme Priesthood Authority

Priest (Houngan) or **Priestess** (Mambo)

Initiate (Hounsis): Initiated into tradition of a particular Loa

Kanzo: Worshipper of the religion

Within its teachings Voodoo has three levels, namely;

Gran Met, Loa's, and the Dead (Note: Language of the Dead). The Gran Met (or rather Grand Master) is named Bondye, a free spirit – able to roam across all plains of existence. Loa's are connected to the 'Mysteries' and are considered to be the ancestral spirits. The Dead is the term used for the 'collective' ancestral spirits that are all around us.

TEACHINGS OF VOODOO:

Gran Met: Grand Master - Architect

Loa: Ancestral Spirits - Knowledge of the Mysteries

The Dead: The Collective - Spirits that are all around us

LOA IDENTITIES:

Erzuli: The Goddess – Protector

Damballah: The Serpent – His companion is Ayida

Ayida Wedo: Beams of light: form of a rainbow – She is with Damballah

Agwe: Sea Creature - Ruler of the Oceans

Ogoun : Battle Dress - A Warrior of the Mysteries

Baron Samedi: Skeleton with a top hat – Loa of the Dead

Ayizan: Human Form - The first Priestess of Voodoo (The First Mambo)

Legba: Guardian of Gates – Note honour him to gain admission

Marassa: The first man and woman – in Union as one (Note: Symbol)

There are three groups that Loa's will be in, such groups will determine if the are malevolent of beneficent spirits:

LOA GROUPS:

Rada – Beneficent: Erzuli, Damballah, Ayida Wedo

Petro – Malevolent: Agwe, Ogoun, Baron Samedi

Ghede – Spirits of the Dead: Ayizan, Legba, Marassa

TYPES OF MAGICAL PRACTICE:

Wanga: Used for protection: Blessing of Charms and creation of Mojo Bags

Veve (Vayv): Powdered eggshell marked upon the ground to create the sacred space – When raising a Loa or Spirits

STRUCTURE OF VOODOO AND ITS ASSOCIATIONS TO THE SERPENT PRIESTHOOD:

BONDYE GRAND MASTER & MISTRESS:

(Not worshipped on the earthly Plain). Associated with the Architect of the Universe in Form; Nammu sometimes referred to as Ilu – as the G.o.d – The Universe complete – He is she and she is he – In union as the life force of existence. There are teachings applied to this aspect of the Trinity.

LOA/DEMON

(Gallas) – Note that Demon practice can be good or bad. Associated with the Eight Points of perfection; note that there are nine Loa Identities, which will lead us in future development towards the Ninth Gate. There are teachings applied to this aspect of the Trinity.

THE DEAD COLLECTIVE ANCESTRAL SPIRITS

Associated with the 'Gidim' – Spirits of the Deep, we have already explored aspects of the Gidim – Our very own transition towards the Ninth Gate. There are teachings applied to this aspect of the Trinity.

ASOGWE (SERPENT PRIESTHOOD)

Supreme Priesthood Authority. Masked over centuries by many names – The ultimate result will lead us to one who is not just with the Serpent, but is further the Serpent in Union.

PRIEST (HOUNGAN) OR PRIESTESS (MAMBO)

Installed into the Serpent priesthood

INITIATE (HOUNSIS)

Initiated into tradition of a particular Loa
As we venture toward the studies of the Eight Points of Perfection we will come to understand the purpose of the eight points and how such points will enlighten us with the K.e.y of our own Magical Abilities

KANZO WORSHIPPER OF THE RELIGION

This is where the fundamental difference occurs. Remember the earlier teachings, as one does not 'worship' as such. To worship would suggest that one would need to be subservient. We know that the Priesthood does not worship, but rather absorbs, embraces. Therefore, one must consider that the 'Kanzo' are indeed the recipients of service, yet not installed within the tradition. In other words, one can conclude that every recipient of our services would be classed as a 'Kanzo'.

Within its teachings we know that Voodoo has three levels, namely; Gran Met, Loa's, and the Dead (Note: Language of the Dead):

GRAND MET ARCHITECT: Knowledge
This is the teachings of the Architect; Nammu. The teachings of destiny, taught to those in the highest degrees, it is named Bondye, for free spirits, able to roam across all plains of existence.

LOA: Knowledge of the Mysteries

Loa teachings are connected to the 'Mysteries' and are considered to be the ancestral spirit teachings. The Dead is the term used for the 'collective' ancestral spirits that are all around us.

THE DEAD: The Collective

This is the collective teaching of the 'Language of the D.e.a.d'; how we are able to communicate by adjusting vibration and internal focus.

From this knowledge we come to realise that the Serpent Priesthood teaches the Language of communication and the Mysteries of the Hidden Knowledge (from the Loa). We further come to realise that Architect Knowledge is for those whom have attained the powers of Loa Magic in all forms – Those who have travelled through the Ninth Gate of the Pyramid of Perfection.

Let us explore the magical teachings in greater depth:

Association with Loa Identities: There are nine – The Nine Gates of the Pyramid!

Nammu: Erzuli (or Ezili) The Goddess – Protector

Ilu: Damballah The Serpent – His companion is Ayida

Amalug: Ayida Wedo Beams of light: Rainbow, She is with Damballah

Mulan: Agwe Sea Creature - Ruler of the Oceans

Nabu: Ogoun   Battle Dress. A Warrior of the Mysteries

Hidden Knowledge: Baron Samedi Skeleton with a top hat. Loa of the Dead

Ansar: Ayizan Human Form. The first Priestess of Voodoo (First Mambo)

Rakbu: Legba Guardian of Gates. Note: honour to gain admission

The Ninth Gate: Marassa First man and woman In Union as one (Note: Symbol)

We now know that there are three groups that Loa's will be in, and that they all have direct associations to the Serpent Priesthood:

Let us now explore the common threads of Voodoo, so to enlighten our minds with the Loa, the Deities:

Marassa (Ninth Gate – Pure Light)

Marassa is 'unusual' in that this divine energy is both considered a Loa, yet abstract within the saddled shores of time. As ancient children in union, Love, Truth, and Justice are the Key to Marassa. We are directed by the links between our world and the world of immortality. In union, these children are able to guide us through the stomach, the sacred Number of 3 in raw state. However, in true form the number of the universal code and language is 1.

Colours: Black, White, and Red

Erzuli (Nammu – Architect)

Erzuli is often referred to as 'Erzulie'; as a wife of Ogoun, Damballah and Agwe, she wears three rings of commitment. She is the scarred woman with a child in one hand, and a knife in the other. She is known by many religions as the 'Black Madonna'; the shadow of Mary Magdalene that will show 'the way'. However, one must remember that Mary is of the Goddess Amalug.

Colours: Navy Blue, Red

Damballah (Ilu – Within)

As a serpent he is considered the 'father' of all Loa. The spiritual home of Loa is known as 'Ginen' and Sacred Rites often enact the stories of Damballah carrying the ancestors back to Ginen. Offerings to Damballah are eggs shells and flour. However, Camphor, Sulphur Brimstone, Salt Petre, and White Crushed Wax are better when creating potions of immortality.

Colour: White

Ayida Wedo (Amalug – Without)

Ayida Wedo is sometimes referred to as 'Aido Quedo' and is associated with rainbows and snakes; hence the term 'Rainbow Serpent'.

Colours: Navy Blue, Red and White

Agwe (Mulan – Insight)

Agwe is the Guardian of the Sea in this world and the 'Sea of Chaos'. If presented with offerings; he will protect the waters of life. His offerings are made by floating 'white willow bark' upon a hand made raft and set upon the waters (oceans, river, stream, or lake)

Colour: Navy Blue

Ogoun (Nabu – Life)

Mighty and powerful would be two words to describe this Deity. The key strengths are with magic and Prophecy. It is said that those whom seek the path of light walk in the shadows of Ogoun. As a warrior, the strength can be channelled into metal tools and weapons.

Colour: Brown

Baron Samedi (Hidden Knowledge – Pyramid)

As a Loa of the Dead he is pictured as a skeleton with a white (or black) top hat, black eyes and a black tuxedo. It is interesting that when translate 'Samedi' means Saturday, as we know Saturday is also the Holy day of the Serpent Priesthood. The Baron will wait at the crossroads to show the way to Ginen (the spiritual land)

Colours: Black, White

Ayizan (Ansar – Magic)

Associated with Voodoo Rites of Installation, and considered to have the knowledge of Priesthood within the Earthly Plain. The working tool used within the installation would be the 'Spirit Rattle'

Colours: White, Yellow, and Gold

Legba (Rakbu – Magic)

Legba lies at the entrance to communication with the spiritual plain. Legba is always the first and last to be called at any Ritual, as he is the voice of G.o.d when opening and closing the Veil. If you are careless, he will trick you to cross the Veil and deny your return therefore, it is important to remind ourselves of the respect we need to provide to Deity. **Colour: Navy Blue**

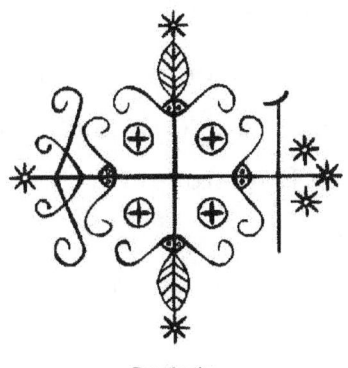

Papa Legba

Now that we have explored the Loa – We must venture to the practice of Opening and Closing a 'Voodoo Ritual':

Voodoo Ritual: To receive assistance from the Loa. This ritual is typical when assistance is required from the Loa. You will need the guidance of all Loa.

Guidance:

- You will need powdered egg shells and white salt combined to seal your Sacred Space
- Place a reciprocal (or cauldron) in the centre of the space
- A light of wisdom to be placed at the centre (These can be candles or tea lights)
- Sulphur Brimstone, Salt Petre, Egg Shell (for Reciprocal)
- Eucalyptus, for the Master of the Swamp (Nabu)
- Smokey Quartz (Ilu) and Tourmaline (Amalug)
- Olive Oil, for Blessing
- Sage, Camphor, and Agrimony mix (Architect, God, and Goddess)
- The Symbol of Papa Legba
- A virgin piece of paper for writing your wish or thoughts

- ⏱ Your Voodoo Doll
- ⏱ Chalice with Holy Water
- ⏱   Red Wine

Sprinkle White Salt and Egg Shell around the Sacred Space, and then light the candle

I ask Legba (Rakbu), Guardian of the Barrier: Protect from malevolent spirits and guide me to the answers I seek

Burn the Sigil of Papa Legba inside the Cauldron – Then sprinkle Sulphur Brimstone into the Cauldron

I give praise and thanks to the Master of the Swamp (Nabu)

Sprinkle Eucalyptus into the Cauldron

Blessed am I to be within the entrance, In the name of Damballah Wedo, Damballah the great, Damballah Lele, Ayida Wedo, Ago, Ago si, Ago La

Anoint yourself with Olive Oil – In the sign of Marassa

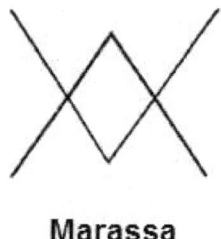

Marassa

I call Agwe (Mulan), Ayizan (Ansar), and Baron Samedi (Hidden Knowledge) to this space to provide insight to me

Sprinkle Salt Petre into the Cauldron

I call Erzuli (Nammu), Damballah (Ilu), and Ayida Wedo (Amalug) to this space to provide protection from within and without

Sprinkle the 'combined potion' (Sage, Camphor, and Agrimony) into the cauldron Then Pour the Holy Water into the Chalice

By the Power of St. Anthony of Padua, Legba Atibon, guardian of the crossroads, Legba guardian of the bush, Legba guardian of the goose; Ago, Ago, Si, Ago La

Drink from the Chalice (The Cup of Life), and then add a small amount of red wine to the Chalice, and say:

Gator Geude, le bon ton roulette, ye, ye, ye

Drink from the Chalice (The Cup of Life)

By the power of the Mistress Erzuli, mamou lade, mamou Vodun, Erzulie Frieda Dahomey, Ago, Ago, Si, Ago. Mamou lade, vie en cane Creole

Be Gone Loa, with peace in mind, I ask Legba (Rakbu), Guardian of the Barrier: Protect from malevolent spirits and close this Veil

Extinguish the Candle

You may now use the potion to throw to the fire, keep in a sealed container and bury in the ground, or add to the sage smudge stick within a Voodoo Doll

HOW TO MAKE (AND USE) A VOODOO DOLL

Items Required to Make Your Doll

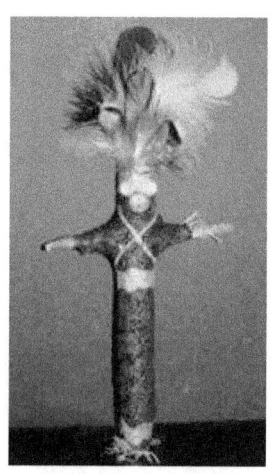

Sage Smudge Stick, two thin small sticks, fabric in 2 inch strips (2/3 feet long of your colour choice), String, 2 small beads (for eyes), a small gemstone of choosing (for mouth), All purpose glue, A box of Map Pins, *Your Loa Assistance Potion (Optional)

> **Warning:** Be careful what you wish for. When we use this level of Magic, we must be certain that it is really what we want to do and achieve. As you have been instructed, you are the only judge within this domain. Please take time to think about why you are going to do, what you are going to do. The effects of this level of Magic are difficult to reverse

Use of Coloured Map Pins:
Black – Repel Negative energy (Send back to sender)
White – Positive energies (enhance to level)
Red – Power

Green – Wealth

Purple – Spirituality

Yellow – Success

Orange – Dream Walkers

Blue – Love and Protection

**Items to use to represent yourself, or
another:** Photograph, used small piece
of clothing, or hair from a brush (always
good to use)

Make your cross with thin sticks: With
your two 'thin' sticks, make a cross –
Then tie them together, bind then with
string

Bind the Sage Padding

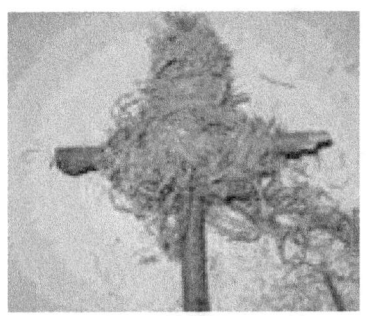

Wrap your Sage Smudge Stick around the Cross. Start at the middle, then down one arm & back to the middle; once the top is complete, work down to the bottom. When you reach the bottom, secure with a piece of ribbon (sellotape can be used).

Bind the material around

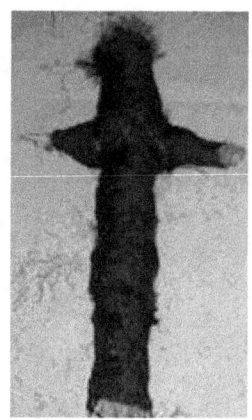

Wrap your material over the Smudge Stick, working around the doll. Start at the middle, then down one arm, then back to the middle. Once the top is complete, work down to the bottom. When you reach the bottom, secure with a piece of ribbon. (secure all together with a small piece of sellotape temporarily) Leave sage for hair and arms

Make the Face

You now need to make the eyes and mouth, with the two beads for the eyes and a small gemstone of your choosing for the mouth. You may wish to consider painting the face on. The face is entirely your personal preference

Add a Pouch and Customise your Doll

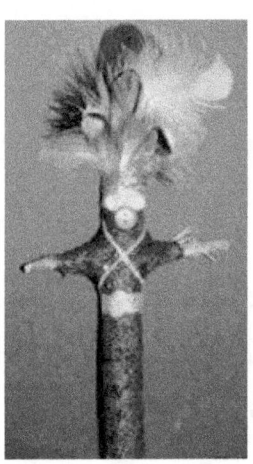

You will need to add a small pouch to hold the personal item(s). You can customise your dolls by adding feathers to the head, creating a headband with ribbon, even a ribbon around the waist. You may consider the doll to carry a Mojo bag, it is entirely personal choice

Cleanse your Doll: You need to cleanse your Doll. Cleanse your hands in Holy Water (as you have been instructed previously). Now work your hand around the doll, saying these words: *Urru annu da A dimmu antam, keezh annu Arazu be Gi ma Dag, wur damu ma bar. Bana gankankha ina Ara ma ina ina zagdaku*

How to Use your Voodoo Doll:

You can use your doll in a variety of ways. For this particular lecture, we will be using the power of 'Thought' to create the magical energy for yourself, collect each of the coloured pins (as previously identified). Light a candle and take a few moments to focus on what it is you wish from each pin for yourself. When ready, place the pin into the Chest of your Doll. As this doll is being used for yourself at this time, you may leave the pins in for as long as you wish. Generally speaking, when using A Voodoo Doll for 'issues' of another person, you must leave the pins in the doll overnight

Be sure to cleanse the Doll every time you remove the pins. Never allow someone else to use your Doll – It is very personal to you

Using your Voodoo Doll – Against another

The most effective way to use your Doll against another is to use the 'doll pouch' for the personal item(s) or photograph in the same way as before. However, this time cleanse the doll as usual, BUT say these words:

Gi ma dara ma salmu ak dag, Neru Ara ina sudal Silig tia altar ina Ara tia Hurapu, Ma zu tia pal ina Gisla Shinar Lah Nigsisa er annu da Ig.igi, Kima A Ak da – Adullab Lipis dir

Night and Dark and Black of Day, Scatter Time in Far Away Hand of mighty in time of lamb, But know of curse in silent land Bring justice to this with those who see, as I do with – Now inwards be

Use of Coloured Pins against another

Black – Send Negative energy (Psychic Attack)

White – Reduce energy (Reduce level)

Red – Diminish Power

Green – Starve Wealth

Purple – Block Spirituality

Yellow – Halt Success

Orange – Dream Walkers

Blue – Blood Magic

How to Make (and use) Mojo Creations

First of all let us indentify what a Mojo Bag is. Over the years, many ideas and beliefs surrounding Mojo have leaped over the realms of reality and truth. Generally speaking, if your life, universe, and everything is looking good for you –Then it could be said that your 'Mojo' is working. But what does this all really mean? Mojo Bags are the best way to describe the powers of energies that live within us, travel through us, and are all around us. It is the very nature of the magnetic forces that 'customise' what we believe, what we see, what we feel, and what we do.

We know that the African tribes have used Mojo creations over the centuries, with a fixed and steady term of 'Wanga', and has been referred to as the 'secret light' – Oftentimes spelt as 'oanga' or 'wanger'. The Wanga is firstly used for protection. However, it does have a multitude of purposes, often installed into the blessing of charms of small potion bags containing herbs, oils, waters, and other less obvious items.

The less 'obvious' items for making Mojo Bags are Solomon's Seal (High John de Conker), Adam and Eve Root, Nag Champa Incense (cone of stick crushed down into a powder), and crushed candle wax. Mojo Bags are made and contained within a plastic sleeve, a piece of material, or even from a 'pre-made' pouch of your choosing. The important thing to remember with Mojo creations is that it is not the presentation of the Mojo that matters – It is the thought, the Energy, and the Inspiration of its maker that becomes the power, the Magic. In today's world – the first time you make a Mojo Bag, I recommend that you follow the 'how to' guidance:

1 – Items Required to Make Your Mojo Bag

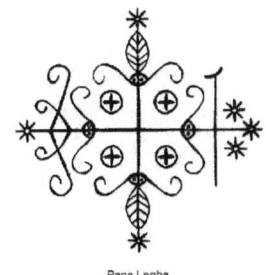

Papa Legba

Plastic bag/sleeve (or piece of cloth), Sigil of Papa Legba, Crushed Candle Wax (Colour of your choosing: See colour chart), Crushed Nag Champa, Kelp, Black Salt, and Crushed Egg Shell, a Tea Light (or standard candle) *Your Loa Assistance Potion (Optional)

> **Warning**: Be careful what you wish for. When we use this level of Magic, we must be certain that it is really what we want to do and achieve. As you have been instructed, you are the only judge within this domain. Please take time to think about why you are going to do, what you are going to do. The effects of this level of Magic are difficult to reverse

Use of Coloured Candles for Positive effect:

Black – Repel Negative energy (Send back to sender)

White – Positive energies (enhance to level)

Red – Power

Green – Wealth

Purple – Spirituality

Yellow – Success

Orange – Dream Walkers

Blue – Love and Protection

Items to use to represent yourself, or

> **another:** Photograph, used small piece
> of clothing, or hair from a brush (always
> good to use)
>
> 2 – Light your candle and Focus

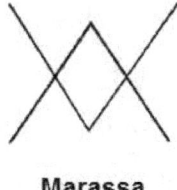

Marassa

Gather your thoughts and feelings, have all your
'items required' around you. Now say these
words:

Urru annu da A dimmu antam, keezh annu Arazu be Gi ma Dag, wur damu ma bar. Bana gankankha ina Ara ma ina ina zagdaku

3 – Add Your Main ingredients

Ayizan

Papa Legba Sigil, Crushed candle Wax (Colour of your choosing: Refer to 'How to'), Crushed Nag Champa Incense, Kelp, Black Salt, Crushed Egg Shell. *Take time to concentrate on your own power of thought whilst mixing the ingredients within you Mojo Bag

4 – Bind Your Mojo

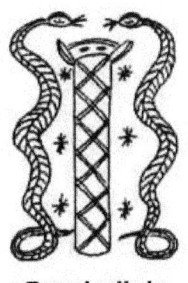

Damballah

Now tie (or seal) your Mojo Bag, this must never be opened again once sealed. Focus once more on what you wish to achieve from the Mojo, and say these words:

A eri da dala ina ara kikig Annu namzu tia kin mimma be

I bind with thorn in time to seek this wisdom of message, whatever to be

5 – Splash hot wax onto your Mojo Bag

Erzuli

With your candle still alight, splash hot wax onto your Mojo Bag, then extinguish the candle

*Your candle must now either be thrown to a fire, or buried within the ground

Your Mojo Creation is now complete: Either bury in the ground with the candle that you used, or throw both to a fire

Using your Mojo Creation Against another:

To use your Mojo Creation against another, replace 'Step 2' words (Light Your Candle and Focus) with:

Gi ma dara ma salmu ak dag, Neru Ara ina sudal Silig tia altar ina Ara tia Hurapu, Ma zu tia pal ina Gisla Shinar Lah Nigsisa er annu da Ig.igi, Kima A Ak da – Adullab Lipis dir

Night and Dark and Black of Day, Scatter Time in Far Away Hand of mighty in time of lamb, But know of curse in silent land Bring justice to this with those who see, as I do with – Now inwards be

Use of Crushed Coloured Candles against another:

Black – Send Negative energy (Psychic Attack)

White – Reduce energy (Reduce level)

Red – Diminish Power

Green – Starve Wealth

Purple – Block Spirituality

Yellow – Halt Success

Orange – Dream Walkers

Blue – Blood Magic

As always, be sure to use this knowledge wisely in your steps towards the Mysteries of Pure Light. Use the hidden knowledge you have received to continue to be steadfast in your practices.

ALCHEMY: A PRACTICAL GUIDE

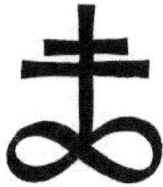

Alchemy is an age-old practice with records dating back to 5000 BCE (to Egyptian Alchemy) and is described as working with natural substances, but further working with the inner-self to transform into higher beings of L.i.g.h.t. The strongest link of the term 'Alchemy' may be sourced from 'al-kimia' (Arabic), meaning 'the art of transformation'.

There are five 'common codes' of Alchemy:

Transmutation: Transformation of metals into gold (known as the 'philosopher's stone'), or transformation of an element into another by reaction.

Panacea (Pay-na-si-a): The formula to cure all illness and prolong life (known as the 'elixir of life') and in oftentimes referred to as the 'water of life'. It should be noted that the name 'Panacea' derives from the Greek healing Goddess.

Spiritual Philosophy: The teachings of spirituality, including mysticism, theosophy, new age reasons, reincarnation, universal mind, and the evolution of the soul. It should be noted that the K.e.y goal of every alchemist is to travel from blindness to enlightenment.

Psychology: The inner meaning of a spiritual path. The practice of alchemy changes the mind and spirit of the individual.

Magnum Opus: (known as 'The Great Work'), having three stages to enlightenment, being; Purification of impurity by the colour of black, enlightenment by the colour white, and unification of the individual with God or rather with the universe).

It is important to recognise that the Magi (the alchemist) does not intend to turn base metals to gold for wealth, but considers the process of transformation to be the very existence of 'testing' the 'elixir of life'. In other words, once the Magi has created a formula, it is added to lead; it is at this very point of reason, that if the substance turns to gold when blended with lead then the 'Elixir' has been found, for life is more precious, far greater, than the materialistic world that consumes the mind. One must consider the K.e.y concepts within the Bible, and how such concepts are riddled with deeper meanings, for example, if we 'adjust' Proverbs 3: 13-20, we discover a altered ego, and altered meaning:

Blessed are those who find wisdom, who gains understanding, for they are more profitable than silver and yield better returns than gold. They are more precious than rubies; nothing you desire can compare with them. Long life is in their right hand; in their left hand are riches and honour. Their ways are pleasant ways, and all their paths are peace. She is a tree of life to those who embrace her; those who lay hold of her will be blessed. By wisdom the Lord laid the earth's foundations, by understanding he set the heavens in place; by his knowledge the deeps were divided, and the clouds let drop the dew. (The Bible, Proverbs 3: 13-20)

If we now re-examine the broken words, we discover that:
1.   By finding wisdom both within (inner-self) and without (all around us), we ar able to see the black flame lit, that which opens the doors of creation to mankind
2.   Once the doors have been open unto us, we are able to tread the path of understanding

3.   It is at the points of reason that we identify with what really matters in the cycle of life, purely life itself, as no material object could succeed in the realms of life and reality. It is therefore the Magi, one who has attained the elixir of life whom achieves wealth, the wealth of the 'hidden knowledge'

4.   The right hand horn sign to be known as a long and fruitful life and in the left hand horn sign, the honour and glory

5.   It is here that we recognise that the path is that of peace, a one world of all worlds, and a universal spirituality

6.   As we embrace the Goddess, we discover that the tree of life was there all along, that the rhythms and codes laid within the foundations open up to those who see

7.   And as we travel from the Goddess to the Lord (or rather the G.o.d of the Northeast), our spiritual awakening occurs and the light of the Southeast, through Earth's foundations is revealed.

Such knowledge understood, divides the spheres of time and embraces the earth and sky; it is here that the creation of the 'water of life' creates a single drop.

We further know that to find the 'Elixir secret', we must further identify with the Emerald tablet, referred to as the 'The Secret of Hermes' – Such tablet is suggested to the secret substance. It is further suggested that Hermes (a Greek God) is identified with the Egyptian God Thoth, making the Emerald Tablet the Tablet of Thoth. The Tablet of Thoth is widely recognised in Alchemy, and Isaac Newton undertook direct translations within his studies of such:

Original Variations of Isaac Newton Translation

1.   It is truth without lying, certainly most true
2.   That which is below is like that which is above, that which is above is like that which is below. To do your miracles on only one thing

3.   All things have been risen by one, by your meditation of One: so all things have their birth by adaptation

4.   The Sun is its father, and the moon its mother

5.   The wind has carried it in its belly, the earth its cradle

6.   The father of all perfection in your world is here

7.   Its force or power is entire if it be converted into earth

8.   Separate this; your earth from your fire

9.   It ascends from your earth to your heaven; again it descends to your earth and receives your force of things superior and inferior

10.   By this means you shall have your glory and your whole world shall fly from you

11.   Its force is above all force, it penetrates every solid thing

12.   So was your world created

13.   Your means and process is here in this

14.   I am called Hermes, having three parts of your philosophy of your whole world

15.   That which I have said of your Sun is accomplished and ended.

The Tablet of Thoth: Meanings and reasons

If we begin to decipher the 'word of words', we begin to see the transformation of the L.i.g.h.t:

1.   Remove all lies to see the Truth

2.   The 'above' and the 'below' are one and the same.

3.   The power of collective thought is sacred – All things will be born by this process

4.   The sun and moon must be in union for enlightenment

5.   The wind is the breath of life, it will nurture

6.   Perfection is within your world, man must make it so

7.   The cycle of life is by converting earth

8.   Separate the soul from the earthly body

9.   Possess the ability to ascend and further to descend

10.   With this understanding you will be transformed

11.   The ability to transform will awaken your within

12.   The earthly plain was created with this knowledge

13.   The process of knowledge is within this

14.   There are three parts to this process

15.   Your sun has become a father and therefore the need of purpose is no more

With the absorption of wisdom and knowledge contained within the Tablet of Thoth, let us explore the 'awakening' with deeper meaning: To awaken the Inner L.i.g.h.t. Let us explore the alchemical transformation, the transformation of deceased to provide life.

Ritual Tools and items required:
A sealed container,
Ground earth (soil),
Air of East - Dried Rose Petals,
South of Fire – Salt Petre,
West of Water - (Holy Water),

Dead matter (Dried Leafs / herbs) – You may choose

Charging Holy Water:

Urru annu da A dimmu antam, Keezh annu Arazu be Gi ma Dag, wur damu ma bar. Bana gankankha ina Ara ma ina ina zagdaku

Guard this gift I order the universe, under this prayer to be night and day, wisdom child and seat of wisdom. Exorcise this vessel in time and in the dark threshold

First Stage:

Place the soil into the container and say:
I place this dirt into the cauldron as a bed for the seeds. Gracious Goddess, bless this Earth that it may bring forth abundance.

Place the Dried Rose Petals into the container and say:

I place dried petal into the cauldron that the smell will remind us of the changing winds that stir up life. Gracious Goddess, bless this Air that it may bring about change for growth.

Place the Salt Petre into the container and say:
I place Salt Petre into the cauldron to fire up the energy lying dormant. Gracious Goddess, bless this Fire that it may release stored energy.

Pour Holy Water into the container and say:
I pour water into the cauldron to dissolve and transmute the materials within, ever remembering that water is life and is the lifeblood of the Mother. Gracious Goddess, bless this Water that may truly be the Universal Solvent.

Stir the potion and say:

I stir this cauldron that the elements within be
mixed, that they may combine and exchange
essences in order that our work be done.
Gracious Goddess, bless our work tonight. And as
the elements transmute to another form, grant
that we also be transmuted into a greater form.

Second Stage:
Place the potion into you container and fill the
container half way, to a maximum of two thirds
Write an action or condition to be transmuted on
a slip of paper, then fold the paper in half and
charge the paper (in the same way as water is
charged). Place the paper into the container with
your potion. It must now remain inside the
container.

Third Stage:
Other items that may be added to your potion at
a later date are:

Hair, nail clippings, blood, semen or other personal items, Ashes from fires, especially from the Yule fire, a small amount of candle wax, or incense (especially Nag Champa). Or even a small amount of crushed eggshell.

Fourth Stage:

You may now seal your jar – It must not be opened again, dripping candle wax onto the edge of the seal will be a good reminder not to open the container again.

You may now cast your potion to water (ocean, stream, or lake), or keep until the next festival, or even bury within the ground.

SYMBOLS OF ALCHEMY:

Within Templar magical practices symbology always plays an important role; symbols that allow one to reach a similarity and conclusion of divine existence. So therefore it is most suiting that we now explore the use of symbols within the first level of the earthly plain and the secondary level of the universe.

Alchemic symbols were devised and introduced as part of the protoscience of alchemy (Philosophical disciplines of Alchemy) and were used to identify elements and compounds. It is important to recognise that symbols and certain styles vary between alchemists. However, there is a 'common thread' in the belief of 'three primes'.

Three Primes:

Most alchemists believe in the concept of the four elements, and that the universe is based upon a 'secondary level', that being three spiritual substances: the 'tria prima' of Mercury, Sulphur and Salt.

Mercury: Transformative agent (fusibility and volatility)

Sulphur: Binding agent between substance and transformation (flammability)

Salt: Solidifying (substantiating) agent (fixity and incombustibility)

And the 'tria prima' defines human identity:

Mercury: Represents the spirit (imagination, moral judgment, higher understanding)

Sulphur: Embodies the soul (emotions and desires)

Salt: Represents the body

The Three Primes

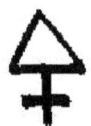 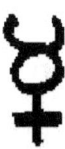 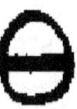

Sulphur   Mercury   Salt

The belief system of three primes, being the spiritual existence of the universe, and further the identity of the soul, being the inward process (of within) and the outward process all around us (the without)

Note: That Sulphur is the G.o.d and Goddess in union, so representing the Triangle (blade) of the G.o.d and the Cross (Equal Space) of the Goddess

One may suggest that if we understand the chemical nature of the 'tria prima', we may discover the nature of all things, so to increase our lifespan. But what does this really mean? Is there life beyond the physical plain of existence? It is important to recognise that the term of 'life' has far spanned the reach of the points of reason. For example, when a living creature ceases to be no more within the earthly plain, do they travel towards a 'new life' from beyond the grave? Simply no; the answer to the existence of life is life itself. Therefore the terms applied to this higher level of consciousness is considered to be 'Ascended' or 'Ascension'.

Let us explore the components of the Trinity in further details, the three primes:

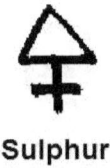

Sulphur

Goddess – Spirit of Life

Sulphur (oftentimes referred to as Brimstone) is an essential element of life, having 'amino acids', and is often referred to a smelling like the dwelling of the modern Christian concept of 'hell', this is far removed, in fact, this sacred powder is used to awaken the senses and aid communication with the Goddess herself. Largely used in fertilizers, matches, and gunpowder, it is a substance that should be handled with care and respect. Locations of Sulphur can be found in Wales, America, Afghanistan, Iran, China, Japan, Russia, Australia, and New Zealand. The best source is from England (in particular; Wadebridge, Cornwall).

Should be handled in small portions and with care.

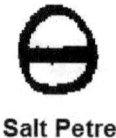

Salt Petre

Green Man – Base Matter

Saltpetre is also known as 'Salt Petre', form Latin, meaning; Stone Salt. Its chemical name is 'Potassium Nitrate', and has been used as an ingredient of fertilizer, smoke bombs, and gunpowder.

Should be handled in small portions, and with care

Mercury

Star – Connection between High and Low (Marshmallow)

A heavy, silvery metal, mercury is one of five metals that are liquid at or near room temperature and pressure. Mercury was known to the ancient Chinese and was transmutation of impure metals into gold. It is a rare element in the Earth's crust. However, it is important to recognise that as previously instructed, substitute with the ingredient Marshmallow leaf. Marshmallow is a member of the hollyhock family. In times past the gum was extracted from the root and processed into sugars as a sweetener for candy.

(Please refer to the complete Sacred Stone and Herb listings for further info on Sulphur, Mercury and Salt.

We now see the Trinity as being:

White (Amalug)   Sulphur – Of the Goddess

Red (Nabu)   Salt Petre – Of the Green Man

Black   Marshmallow – Of the Future Star
(Mulan)

By identifying with the symbols of alchemy, we have further discovered that the G.o.d and the Goddess are now in 'union' with the blade of the G.o.d and the cross of the Goddess combined, creating the true symbol of the Goddess:

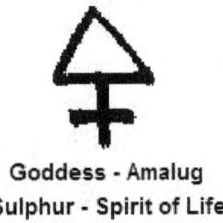

Goddess - Amalug
Sulphur - Spirit of Life

We further identify with the Path of L.i.g.h.t, the 'Future Goddess Star', and the recognition that the marshmallow is used within the Trinity for the future star:

<u>Future Goddess Star - The True Trinity</u>

<u>Southeast</u>	<u>North</u>	<u>Southwest</u>
Black Spirits	**White Spirits**	**Red Spirits**
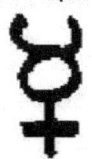	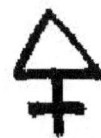	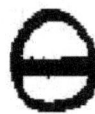
Star - Mulan	**Goddess - Amalug**	**Green Man - Jul (Nabu)**
Marshmallow - Connection	**Sulphur - Spirit of Life**	**Salt Petre - Base Matter**
Wand	Sword	Chalice

Note: The transit of the G.o.d and the Goddess in union arrives in the North, the point of the ascended triangle

We will continue by identifying with the planetary symbols and how such symbols relate to the seven base metals and planets:

The Planetary Symbols of Alchemy

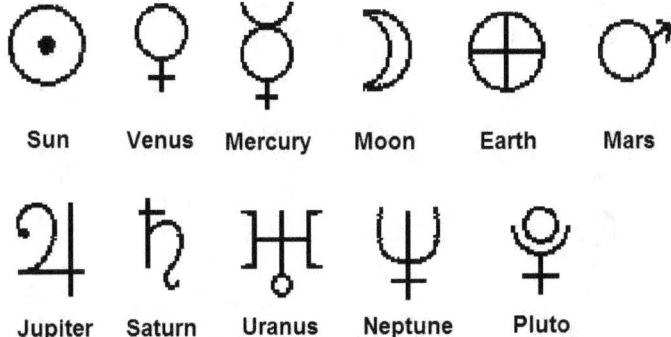

Sun   Venus   Mercury   Moon   Earth   Mars

Jupiter   Saturn   Uranus   Neptune   Pluto

'It was 2029 when first contact occurred'

The Seven Base Metals and their Planetary Association

☉
Sun
Gold — Healing, Protection, Wisdom

☽
Moon
Silver — Psychic Ability, Invocation, Peace

♀
Venus
Copper — Luck, Healing, Energy

♂
Mars
Iron — Cleansing, Focus, Insight

♃
Jupiter
Tin — Awareness, Stability, Direction

☿
Mercury
Mercury — Enlightenment, Progression

♄
Saturn
Lead — Inner Knowledge, Realisation

The Philosopher's Stone

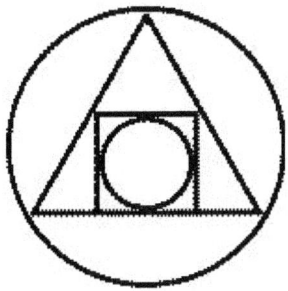

As you will note below, this specific alphabet is the very basis of existence within the universe as one; trails of the association with these symbols span across several belief systems and in particular may be traced through many magical talismans. The K.e.y to focus upon here within these studies are the letters: A, M, N, P, Q, W, Y, and I.

The Alphabet in Alchemy:

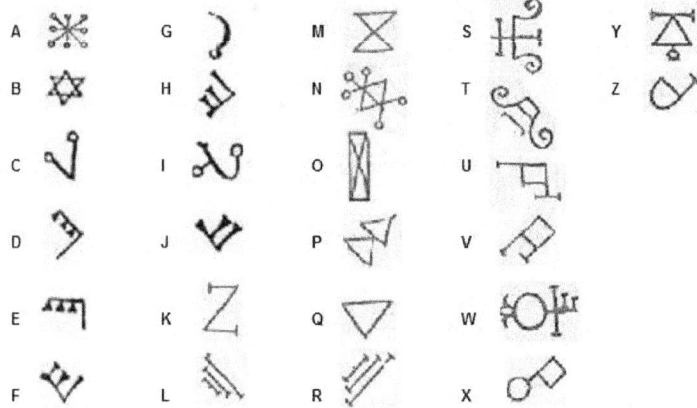

The alphabet symbols are considered 'sacred symbols' within Gnostic Orders and in particular; can be best applied during the alchemical transformation of the Benu Bird (or rather the Phoenix). The Benu Bird is associated with the three energies, named in Egypt as Atum, Re, and Osiris. The Benu Bird is said to have flown high above the waters of creation, then came to rest upon the rock of truth, and at this perfect point in time it brought life and L.i.g.h.t into the world. Its life was fulfilled for five hundred years, then upon the point of death it was set alight with a mix of herbs and Sacred symbols. From the ashes a new Benu Bird would be born.

It is of no surprise that the Benu Bird bears similar tales to that of the Phoenix. The phoenix moulds myrrh into an egg shape and hollows out the centre, places its father and sacred symbols into the centre, then seals the opening with myrrh. Once the perfection of the shape is complete, the Phoenix buries the egg in the 'Temple of the Sun' in Egypt, and it is at this perfect point that the Phoenix is reborn through the process of alchemical transformation. So to understand the initial phase of existence, we must venture through our 'Rites of Passage' by performing a working from the 'Egyptian Book of the Dead' – so to experience (for a short period of time) the awakening of the phoenix with the knowledge of the past life.

'Seek not those whom choose a path of security, but rather find those whom will inspire and challenge every thought you have been programmed with'

THE ALCHEMICAL TRANSFORMATION – INITIAL PHASE:

You will need:
Two Pieces of Virgin paper,
A Candle,
Myrrh,
Holy Water (Charged water, as previously instructed),
Reciprocal

Chose two of the Symbols from the Alphabet – being; A, M, N. P. Q, W, Y, or I

Now draw one symbol on each of your pieces of paper:

Light the candle and focus upon the flame – when ready place both your pieces of paper to the flame

Now speak the Word of Words below:

I have flown up like the primeval ones

I have become Khepri

I have grown as a plant

I have clad myself as a tortoise

I am the essence of every God

I am the seventh of those seven Uraei who came into being in the West

Horus who makes the brightness with his person

That God who was against Seth

Thoth who was among you in that judgement of Him who presides over Letopolis together with the Souls of Heliopolis, The flood which was between them

I have come on the day when I appear in glory with the strides of the gods

For I am Khons who subdued the Lords

As for him who knows this pure spell

It means going out into the day after death and being transformed at will, being in the suite of Wennefer

Being content with the food of Osiris

Having invocation offerings
Seeing the sun; It means being hale on earth
with Re and being vindicated with Osiris, and
nothing evil shall have power over him
A matter a million times true.

Extinguish the Flame.

'For when the riddles of time do stand the wager
in a mighty hand -/-

POTION PREPARATIONS, POUCHES AND CANDLES:

TEMPLAR POTIONS:

At this, the stage of the Templar Potions being revealed, it is of utmost importance to give time to yourself to fully absorb the knowledge given to the making of the Templar Potions.

How to use your Potion

There are three distinct ways to use this Sacred Potion:

a) Mix with Olive Oil into a paste for the powers of healing; or

b) Take a moments thought in a quiet place – use your own power of thought with a candle alight and focus upon the 'here and now' – When it feels right to do so; blow out the candle and throw the potion to an open fire; or

c) Mix with olive oil and water within an 'oil burner' and relax in the knowledge that the energies contained within will fill your chosen space

A student's guide for creating potions, pouches, candles and lotions etc:

With all of the above knowledge now firmly in place, you are able to draw upon this wisdom to create potions, lotions, spells, pouches, candles etc of your own choosing and desire.

Alchemy and magic is an Art of beauty; often know as The Black Arts, and must always be used wisely and responsibly with your uppermost outcome always placed truly in mind. Here are few working recipes, as an example to provide a starting point in time, as way of a kick-start for any student:

Aches, Pains and Bruising:

Combine Frankincense, Kelp and White Willow – grind well in a pestle and mortar and mix to a lotion with olive oil. Massage gently into affected areas.

Ankle and Knee Rub:

Combine Sulphur Brimstone, White Willow Bark and Mugwort; grind well into a paste with olive oil and apply to affected areas

Anti – biotic and Anti – inflammatory:

Combine well in a pestle and mortar: Burdock (anti-inflammatory), Sage (anti-biotic), Wormwood (anti- bacterial) Mix together with olive oil and use as a poultice on affected areas. Also good as a lotion applied to insect bites and stings

Beltane Offering to Inanna:

Combine White Willow Bark, Burdock Root and Lavender – offer in a pouch or sprinkle during rite. May be added carefully to a tea-light or as an anointing potion in candle magic.

Body Lotion:

Combine 3 of the following: Frankincense, Lilly Leaf, Marjoram or Marigold. Grind well in a pestle and mortar and mix to a lotion with olive oil. Apply as a lotion to body.

Cleansing of Chapel, Lodge or Preceptory
Smoulder Honeysuckle and Eucalyptus in a cauldron with Clear Quartz; leave until the next meeting and use again.

Cleansing of Spirit Board for Personal and Singular Use:
Use Rosemary, Hops and Marigold mixed in water on the board.

Dental Treatment (support during)
Take with you, a pouch containing Lavender, a piece each of serpentine, obsidian and Amethyst. On arriving home place the Lavender into a small fire alight and pause in a moment of thought on health and well-being.

Dream Travel:

Combine Holly Leaf, Mugwort and Mullein – grind in a pestle and mortar, add to a pouch and place under your pillow or can be added carefully to tea-light or as an anointing potion in candle magic

Energy, Inspiration and Clarity:
Combine Lavender, Eucalyptus and White Sage – wear in a pouch on your person or leave under your pillow at night. Can be added carefully to tea-light or as an anointing potion in candle magic

Face Lotion for soft skin and anti-wrinkles:
Combine Frankincense, Lilly Leaf and Holly Leaf – grind well in a pestle and mortar and mix together in a paste with olive oil.

Face Wash:
Make up a mixture of Kelp in water for physical perfection.

Intellectual Achievements and Focussing the Mind.

Place in a pouch – Tiger Eye (focussing the mind), Rosemary (intellectual achievement), Raspberry Leaf (focussing the mind), Mullein Leaf (clarity, good luck and mental focus)
Wear as a pouch or pendant, place under your pillow or hang in the home.

Important Occasions such as Exams etc:

Use a combination of Mullein Leaf: (To banish negativity, to promote good luck, for mental focus, for clarity and insight). Lavender: (For expansion of consciousness, for stimulation of physic powers, to aid meditation, for inspiration and mental control). Raspberry: (For focussing the mind, protection during travel and visualisation)
Wear in a pouch on your person or leave under your pillow at night; can be added carefully to a tea-light or as an anointing potion in candle magic. May also be hung around the home in a pouch.

Itchy Areas of Skin:

Combine Wormwood, Burdock Root, Solomon's Seal; crush and make into a paste with olive oil and apply to affected areas

Loa Potion: for Magical Uses and Mojo Bags

Combine Sage, Camphor and Agrimony

Massage Paste:

Combine 3 of the following – Marshmallow Leaf, Camphor, Raspberry Leaf, Rosemary – grind well in a pestle and mortar and mix to a paste with olive oil and use on affected areas.

Massage Oil to Comfort and Re-energise:

Combine Frankincense (for re-energising areas of the body), White Willow Bark (For calming pain), Sulphur Brimstone (for muscle aches) use sparingly. Mix well in a pestle and mortar and combine into a massage lotion with olive oil.

Massage Oil for Feet and Bones:

Combine Apple Leaf (re-alignment of energy and bones) with White Willow Bark (For calming pain) Mix well into a massage lotion with olive oil and massage given areas.

Massage Paste for Tired, Aching Muscles:

Combine Mugwort (tired muscles and rheumatism), White Willow Bark (For calming pain), Sulphur Brimstone – sparingly (For muscle aches). Grind together and mix to a paste with olive oil and apply to sore, aching joints.

Mouthwash/Rinse for Gums:

Agrimony – mix with water and use as mouthwash.

Myrrh – gargle with, as above.

Thyme, Mint and Cinnamon – soak in water for five weeks, drain and use as a mouthwash.

Muscle Spasm and Inflammation:

Combine 3 of the following; Solomon's Seal, Kelp, Honeysuckle and White Willow Bark in a pestle and mortar, grin finely and add to olive oil to make a lotion. Apply to affected areas.

Protection:

1. Sprinkle Marjoram, Mint and Rosemary in or around a given area for protection.
2. Sprinkle Black Salt and/or Kelp around household or garden boundary for protection.
3. Carry Marshmallow in a sachet for protection.

Re-cleansing of returned working tools:

Charge with holy water, using Adventurine and Clear Quartz in the water. Use the standard script for cleansing stones located in the scriptures given.

Skin Conditions:

Combine Wormwood, Honey Suckle and Solomon's seal or Wormwood, Burdock Root and Solomon's seal or simply Mint and mix well to a paste with olive oil and apply to skin.

CANDLES AND NIGHT-LIGHTS WITHIN THE HOME:

1Protection, Energy, Communication, Dreams and Good Luck: Anoint a Blue Candle with a mixture of Holly Leaf and Hawthorn or sprinkle mixture sparingly into a night-light. (Can be used in combination with Blue Lace Agate and Moonstone)

2Wisdom, Knowledge, Good Fortune, Positive Dreams: Solomon's seal.

3Physic Abilities, Inspiration, Visions, Wisdom: Acacia.

4Banish Negativity, Clarity, Insight, Life Giver, Good Luck: Mullein Leaf.

5Courage, Power, Creativity and Energy, Travel and Strength: Anoint a Red Candle with a mixture of Wormwood and Mugwort or sprinkle sparingly into a tea-light (Use in combination with Carnelian and/or Obsidian)

6Love, General Healing, Rebirth, Peace and Harmony: Anoint a White Candle or sprinkle sparingly into a tea-light (can be used in combination with Lapis lazuli).

7Protection and Energy/ to Block Negativity: Anoint a Yellow Candle with a mix of Sage and Agrimony. (for use in Candle Magic)

8To Drain and Steal Power: Anoint a Black Candle with Mandrake Root and Wormwood (for use in Candle Magic)

9Courage and Energy: Anoint a Red Candle with Mandrake Root and Wormwood (for use in Candle Magic)

EARTH CYCLE POTIONS:

When creating potions for friends and family as gifts etc, one may create more specific combinations that reflect ones own creativity – such as these 'Earth Cycle Potions'. These specially prepared Templar potions can connect each individual to the seasonal cycles and the sacred energies of our planet and can be prepared and made as and when required. THESE POTIONS ARE MAGICALLY CHARGED USING THE 'CHARGING SCRIPT' GIVEN AS PER OUR ANCIENT TEMPLAR KNOWLEDGE AND WISDOM. THEY CAN BE USED AS AN INCENSE, KEPT IN A POUCH, SPRINKLED SPARINGLY IN A LIGHTED TEA-LIGHT OR SPRINKLED IN YOUR BATH WATER OR ABOUT YOUR SURROUNDINGS.

'The Energies of Autumn':

A MAGICALLY CHARGED POTION TO ASSIST YOU
IN ACCESSING YOUR OWN INNER REALMS OF
CONSCIOUSNESS AND EMPOWERMENT:
CREATED OF **WORMWOOD, KELP, DILL AND
MUGWORT** TO CONNECT YOU TO THE Energies
of Autumn.

USE FOR TRAVELLING WITHIN, FOR
CONNECTING TO THE UNDERWORLD AND TO
THE ANCESTRAL SPIRITS, AND FOR INCREASING
PSYCHIC POWERS.

'The Energies of Winter':
A magically charged potion to assist you in
accessing your own inner realms of consciousness
and empowerment: Created of **Burdock Root,
Myrrh, Sage and Solomon's Seal** to connect
you to the Energies of Winter.
Use for discovering your inner depths &
quietness, for accessing the 'within', for
recharging & re-establishing energies, inner
strength & focus.

'The Energies of Spring':
A MAGICALLY CHARGED POTION TO ASSIST YOU
IN ACCESSING YOUR OWN INNER REALMS OF
CONSCIOUSNESS AND EMPOWERMENT:
CREATED OF **HAWTHORN, CAMPHOR, OLIVE
AND APPLE LEAF** FOR CONNECTION TO THE
Energies of Spring,

USE TO UPLIFT THE SPIRIT, RAISE
CONSCIOUSNESS AND ASSIST IN LOVE.

'The Energies of Summer':
A MAGICALLY CHARGED POTION TO ASSIST YOU
IN ACCESSING YOUR OWN INNER REALMS OF
CONSCIOUSNESS AND EMPOWERMENT:
CREATED OF **LAVENDER, APPLE LEAF, ACACIA
AND EUCALYPTUS** TO CONNECT YOU TO THE
Energies of Summer.

USE TO RAISE ENERGY, CREATE ABUNDANCE
AND EXPANSION, FULFILLMENT AND LOVE,
INSPIRATION AND PSYCHIC ABILITIES

Herbal magic, potions, sacred herbal preparations etc, and the magical preparation, charging of potions and compounds are just some of the aspects of Templar Alchemy as taught on the Knight Templar path; taught in the same way as originally taught many aeons ago by the original 'Old Ones'…….

'If you witness a death, you will realise that at the point of death an energy release occurs – BUT, what if you could harness this energy from yourself prior to death?'

THE SCRIPTS AND CHARGES FOR WORKING WITH HERBS, POTIONS AND SACRED STONES:

Cleansing of Water:

Before any kind of magical work, healing or ceremony one must first cleanse the water. To do this you will need to perform a widdershins (anticlockwise) movement around your receptacle of water, your left hand held out flat and knuckles upwards. As you do so recite the following words:

"Urru annu da A dimmu antam, Keezh annu Arazu be Gi ma Dag,
wur damu ma bar. Bana gankankha ina ara ma ina ina zagdaku"

Guard this gift I order the universe,
under this prayer to be night and day,
wisdom child and seat of wisdom.
Exorcise this vessel in time and in the dark threshold.

The water is now cleansed and charged; to be used for cleansing hands prior to workings and for many other magical practices.

Charging the Rakbu Dag or Samnu Emua for Healing Practices:
The following mystical chant can be used for various magical purposes; not solely for charging the boards. Have all stones aligned on the board of your choice, with the appropriate channelling stone in your left hand; knuckles upwards, take time to tune into the energies of the channel board; again travel with a Widdershins motion and when ready recite the Mystic Chant:

*"E-gish-shir-gal, E-gish-shir-gal
Lu Annu bi ma lalartu eri"*

*House of Great Light, House of Great Light,
Let this divide and phantom bind*

After this, your patient/client or you chooses two appropriate stones for the healing treatment. One Stone is chosen for its magical ability and the other stone for its healing abilities. Place both the chosen stones into the chalice of water and with your LEFT hand flat, you can now perform the Script of Ea, again widdershins around the chalice: -

"Nabu Kur Dingar, E ina Utu, Nanna, ma Adar
Su'ati annu Piriq, ina Azag
Annu tisa bi er E Gallas
Mamman aga Azag bur annu aka annu wur eri"

Nabu underworld God, raise the Sun, Moon, and star that this the bearer of the magic, from the shining bright this ninth command to go raise demons. Whoever crowns the shining bright hear this divine command, this wisdom bind

At this point the healing would thus take place; full instruction of which are in this book.

Charging of Herbs and Potions (from the Working of the Dead):

The following script is to be used to charge all prepared herbs, herb sachets or mixed potions, lotions, pastes, candle mixes and spell use of etc, prior to use by yourself in practice or as a gift to others. For this charging you will need the tourmaline taken from a chalice of holy/charged water and with the tourmaline within your grasp and again knuckles upward to the above. Repeat the 'working script" whilst travelling widdershins (anticlockwise) around the prepared herbs.

Kima A gub annu da Keezh ina Arazu tia Ara
Negelta ina walvbane silig
Ina bilga ar ma Adar tia dima zig Alka Aradu es
Arata ma Lu ba es ushum uri ina zid
Ur ma Enlil ma uri ma esentu Qannu tia wur abba
ama Bi annu da tia E'Kur ana

As I cleanse this gift under the prayer of time. Awake from able shepherd's hand. From ancestor light and star of judgement stand. Come descend on Earth and let live on dragon blood in truth Ground and air and blood and bone. Horn of wisdom elder strong Command this gift of high mound one.

The gifts of potions or herbs are now ready for your own use or to pass on to others.

Please Note the following:

10When using Tea-lights, sprinkle sparingly and carefully into liquid wax and allow to cool before using as a gift for others or for ones self. Always extinguish candles before anointing, for candle magic

11All herbs can be substituted with Sage if necessary and Black Salt can be substituted with Kelp.

12Use a combination of 3 potions only until you become proficient in your Art.

13Important – do not use the combinations on broken skin, internally or if you have allergies to any of the above.

.

QANTUM MALA INA KIAM MAL GERIU MAK
Original recipe for true Black Salt

Wulltree mak malun settu sep inka mer, lu mila iamu set kur mana man mer

سوء كانتام ماك جريو العراقية الخيام القانون النموذجي للتحكيم

To formulate such a potent mix can be tiresome, yet adventurous at the exact moment in time. One may consider the first question as to WHY you feel the need (or wish) to create a form of Magi potion. Is it for good? Is it for protection of yourself or another? Clearly this potent mix which is known in modern times as 'Black Salt' is dangerous within the wrong hands of lore.

One begins to speculate as to why you are reading this? What purpose does it have within your existence? More importantly; what will you learn and actually achieve for concocting such a mix?

If your mind (and heart) is well founded, you may go in peace and prepare this Sacred Potion, bearing in mind the need to use the 'mixture of innocence' with the Magi Code. We mean no harm to any or all. The innocence must be prepared from yourself, the WoRd made FleSH for all to see and know. This is the secret of the potion and only from the nine of Wull within the Tree of Life are we truly able to see the reasoning within reason.

Go far and travel well, go long and travel high, for now is time of creation, and we have but not long within this to create such a creation with this world. You live and breathe within the knowledge of the creation, that Malak and Kiam will soon come to reveal that of revelation. For in time, and without cause this potion will prove to be an amicable opponent within.

Part Flesh i.e. Nail clippings, dried hair, dried ear wax, dried and ground eye lashes

Part Ground Pepper For the age of Time to sea of life

Part Ground Kelp From the non-existence within creation, the opposite of the Earth

Parts Salt May be sea salt, flesh salt, or simple processed salt

'The Granite dispersed and I saw beams of Light emanating from the Earth'

'As the darkness consumed the Earth, terror unfolded through the rays of light'

TO KNOW - TO WILL - TO DARE - TO KEEP SILENT

'Knowledge is gained, and Wisdom attained by degrees. During the earlier stages of the search for truth, it is but natural that the mind is beclouded, and comprehension at a loss. It is during this period that the Neophyte must remember the command: Go forward, have faith and knowledge will unveil itself.'

THE MYSTERY OF MAGIC

The art of magic consists in employing invisible or so-called *Spiritual* agencies, the Hierarchies or Principalities of Light, to obtain visible results.' The term 'Magic' as here used is not to be confused with the general meaning or usage of the word. In the Occult or spiritual application of the word, it indicates the direction of a force in Nature generally unknown. He who in sincerity enters the study of the *Great Work*, at once begins to live a double life. One life he lives in the imitation spirit, as do all men, but he also lives another life in the conscious *Spirit* which through his efforts is being developed. The conscious *Spirit* is the fruit of years of study and training. Man is unknown to himself until he begins to consciously make an effort to find the real self within himself and which allies him to the invisible Spiritual Hierarchies.

Gradually, after studying and long training, he begins to sense the other, the hidden self, and to comprehend the part he plays in the great drama of life. Man cannot *know* God of the *Spiritual* things until he becomes a child of the *Light*. Then, and then only, is his relationship with God established. While man lives only in the imitation spirit, he does not truly live; he exists as the plaything of fate and characters stronger than himself. He is a pawn in the game of life. When he establishes the conscious life, then, the *Light* gives life. He will see life as it is, and irrespective of where he may be, there will be the *Spiritual* forces to command. Like David of old, he can no longer hide from God, for God is everywhere. Almost from the very beginning, the Neophyte is engaged in seeking this *Light* and in connecting with the Hierarchies or Principalities of *Light*, because therein alone is to be found that which is above the human equation. *This does not make him less human or less practical*. It enhances his understanding of the self and his usefulness to his fellow creatures.

This is as far as we are permitted to travel at this point in time; further information on Alchemy, Magic, Sacred Stone and Herbal Practices, the history of the Knight Templar and very much more, which go into greater and deeper depths of knowledge, can be found within the 'Knights Bible' in the context of the Knight Templar degrees; further teachings that travel deeper still towards the truths of existence can be found in the teachings of 'The Sanctuary' and 'The Priory'.

Alternatively please contact the author for further teachings of the Knight Templar path, The Sanctuary and The Priory.

or see

http://www.misterree.com/
http://priory7.wix.com/priory
https://themidnightgarden.wordpress.com/

'When the End arrives, those whom had doubt will no longer'

'The person who hears my words and does nothing with them is like a stupid or foolish man who built his house on the sand'

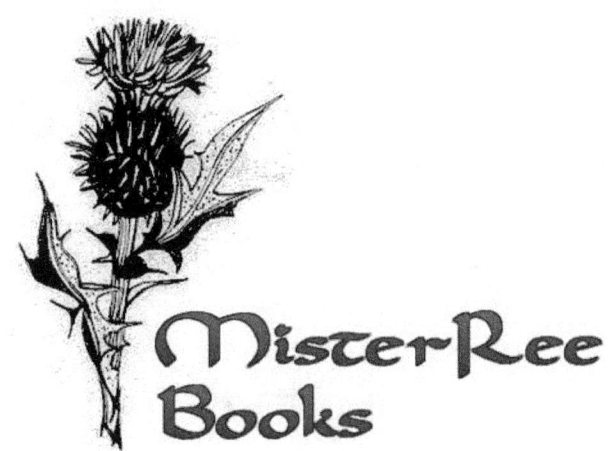

MisterRee Books

Editors Note   K.e.y 1 3

Sbe vg jnf ng gung gvzr gung V ernyvfrq gung gb
gur Cynarg anzrq Rnegu V jbhyq fb geniry. V qvq
abg jnag gb iragher gb fhpu n cynpr ng vg jnf
xabja gung gubfr jubz unq ratvarrerq gur uhznaf
unq perngrq fhpu n perngher gung jbhyq or
svyyrq jvgu terrq naq pbeehcgvba. Vg jnf ng guvf
cbvag bs neeviny gung V erpnyy ubj gur uhznaf
jrer naq jung gurl fubhyq xabj gurl qvq abg. Sbe
nyy gur clenzvqf bs sbeghar jrer fb oheevrq
orarngu gurve anzr bs Rnegu naq fhpu gernfherf
jbhyq bcra gur urneg bs nal perngher fb gb frr vg
vaare ornhgl. Sbe ng gur ryriragu ubhe va gur
Uvtu zbhaq bs gur Vfyr funyy lbh frr gur havdhr
raretl gung qbgu pbzr sebz orybj. Gur Frpbaq
pbzvat vf urer, naq fb hagb guvf jbeyq bs zna
funyy or xabja.

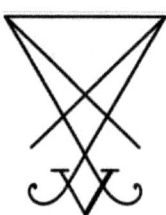

www.ingramcontent.com/pod-product-compliance
Lightning Source LLC
Chambersburg PA
CBHW051441170526
45166CB00001B/70